Mind-Blowing
Orgasms
Every Day

D1526834

Mind-Blowing Orgasms Every Day

365
WILD AND WICKED WAYS TO
REVITALIZE YOUR SEX LIFE

CYNTHIA W. GENTRY

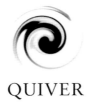

QUIVER

First published in the USA in 2005 by
Fair Winds Press
33 Commercial Street
Gloucester, MA 01930

08 07 06   2 3 4 5

ISBN 1-59233-209-9

Library of Congress Cataloging-in-Publication Data
Gentry, Cynthia W.
   [Bedside orgasm book]
   Mind-blowing orgasms every day : 365 wild and wicked ways to
revitalize your sex life / Cynthia W. Gentry.
      p. cm.
   Originally published: The bedside orgasm book.
   Includes bibliographical references and index.
   ISBN 1-59233-209-9 (alk. paper)
   1. Sex instruction for women. 2. Women--Sexual behavior.
3. Sexual excitement. 4. Orgasm.   I. Title.
HQ46.G46 2006
613.9'6--dc22

                                        2006010578

Cover design by Mary Ann Smith
Book design by Barb Karg
Printed and bound in Singapore

To Nima, my muse

ACKNOWLEDGMENTS

Writing this book has been a surprising, incredible personal and creative journey—and not just because it's supplied me with amazing cocktail party conversation. I am deeply indebted to many, many people for their support. First, I would like to thank my editor Paula Munier, who thought of me for this project and its predecessor. Thanks, Paula, for your faith, patience, and encouragement.

My undying gratitude goes to my agent Sheree Bykofsky and her associate Megan Buckley, whose advice and support saw me through many angst-ridden days. Without them, I probably would have chickened out early on. Thanks as well to Homan Taghdiri, who offered outstanding guidance and counsel.

I'm indebted to the friends and family members who cheered me on. My writing buddy, Susanne Pari, sat across from me at a local café day after day and was always willing to take a break from her own projects to help me with mine. Thaisa Frank, whose input was so valuable for my last book, gave me superb counsel about approaching this one. Thanks, too, to David Ramsdale, who generously shared his expertise and gave me ideas and advice. My mother was, of course, always there when I needed her, even if it took me a while to admit to her the true nature of my latest "writing project."

I also have to thank the many friends, and friends of friends, who responded to me so enthusiastically with their own experiences and tips. I was touched by their candidness and willingness to share the intimate details of their lives with me. I would name them here, but I suspect they'd kill me. Besides, I'm too afraid of leaving someone out.

Nima, my muse, my love, and my truly significant other, never flagged in his love and support, and didn't blink an eye when I brought my computer and a suitcase full of sex books along on a Hawaiian vacation. Thank you for believing in me, even when I didn't. You make it easy for me to love you, twenty-four hours a day, seven days a week, and 365 days a year.

TABLE OF CONTENTS

INTRODUCTION

365 Days (and Nights) of Bedroom Bliss!

Welcome to *Mind-Blowing Orgasms Every Day*! In these pages, you'll find 365 ideas to spice up your love life with innovative sex play, naughty recipes, creative positions from the sex classics, including the *Kama Sutra*, and much, much more. You'll be introduced to the new generation of sex toys (for him and her), given refreshers on basic techniques, and shown how to put the excitement back into standard positions like the Missionary. You'll learn how to tell your partner what you want in ways that are guaranteed to turn him on, not off, and you'll unlock the sensual secrets of deeply satisfying sex.

Whether you're playing alone, trying to reignite the flames in an established marriage, or things are just starting to heat up with a new partner, you'll find plenty of tips and techniques to keep your love life humming. "Position of the Week" spotlights sex positions you'll want to make the basics of your repertory. Shy about masturbation? You won't be once you read these hot tips! (Remember, knowing your own responses is the key to having great orgasms—or, quite often, any orgasms.) Oral and manual sex techniques will show you how to make any man putty in your hands—and keep him coming back for more. And, of course, there are plenty of sensual treats for him to use to drive *you* wild, too!

From how to act out your favorite fantasies to the art of talking dirty (even the suggestion may be enough to fan his flames), how to dress for success and mastering the art of married dating (hint: send the sitter and kids out!) to taking sex out of the bedroom, seducing him at your favorite restaurant, sensual massage and water play, and transforming your bedroom into a love nest, a wealth of sensual delight awaits you in *Mind-Blowing Orgasms Every Day*. Which tip will you try tonight?

CHAPTER ONE

JANUARY

"One kind word can warm three winter months."
—Japanese proverb

The ancient Romans named January after *Janus*, the god of gates and doors—in other words, the god of openings and beginnings. So look at this month as a time for a new sexual beginning, a time to put the past behind you and start the year afresh. Explore the openings not only of your own body, but of your heart and mind as well. Think of January as a month of possibilities, a chance to start out with a clean slate—a clean sexual slate, that is.

This month's birth flowers are *carnations* and *snowdrops*. In Victorian times, a carnation symbolized bonds of affection, as well as pure and deep love. A beautiful snowdrop symbolized hope. Why not keep a vase of fresh carnations and snowdrops in a corner of your bedroom, to symbolize your hopes for a new year of pure ecstasy?

January's birthstone, the deep red *garnet*, is a symbol of constancy and commitment. Buy a garnet-colored candle or other token to remind you that this month, you're committed to pleasure!

JANUARY

Make a List of Ten Sensual Resolutions

This year, let's create a list that will be a pleasure to keep: a list of Ten *Sensual Resolutions*. Your Sensual Resolutions can as naughty, nice, or elaborate as you want. If you can't think of ten, don't worry. If you forget them midway through the year, don't worry about that, either. You can always add to the list later, or even make up a new one. Begin each sentence with "I resolve," and keep the focus positive. For example:

+ I resolve to honor and love my sensual, sexual self as an integral, beautiful part of my being.

+ I resolve to think of myself as a sensual, sexual person, no matter what my age, height or weight!

+ I resolve not to worry too much about whether or not I have an orgasm. Instead, I'll enjoy the sensations and closeness I feel with myself or a partner.

+ I resolve to explore and enjoy my body without shame.

+ I resolve to try at least three new sexual positions this year!

+ I resolve to enact at least one of my sexual fantasies, as long as it's emotionally and physically safe. One fantasy is_____ (describe it here).

+ I resolve to tell my partner what really pleases me.

+ I resolve to buy myself one really fabulous piece of sexy underwear!

+ I resolve to have an orgasm a day!

Remember, these are just suggestions. Your Sensual Resolutions are for your eyes only, unless you decide you really want to share them with a partner. Now that you've written your list, put at least one of your resolutions into practice—today!

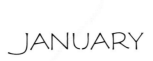

JANUARY

Get to Know Your Gateway to Pleasure

Are you ready to inaugurate your sensual year? In honor of *Janus*, the god of openings, let's take some time to get acquainted with that opening through which all life—and a lot of pleasure—flows: Your vagina. Ladies, it's time to get to know and love your sacred cave.

Get a mirror and lie down on your bed or a couch. Make yourself comfortable. Position the mirror between your legs, and take a look. Enjoy the view—your lover does! Notice the fleshy folds of your *labia majora*, or outer lips, and the hairless inner lips of your *labia minora*. Labia come in all sizes, shapes, and colors, so appreciate the distinctive features of yours just as you might an exotic flower. (Ever seen the Georgia O'Keefe painting *Red Canna*?) You'll also see your clitoral hood and vaginal opening.

Gently stroke the moist folds, and if you'd like, stretch open your lips to caress your vaginal opening. When you're ready, slide one or two fingers inside. Feel the folds and ridges that line the sensitive outer third of your vagina; most of the nerve endings are actually located here. Plunge deeper and deeper into your juicy hole as you imagine a lover thrusting inside you. If at this point, you can't keep your hands off your clitoris, that's fine. Just keep your fingers inside your vagina, and if you can, notice the amazing feelings as you give yourself over to ecstasy!

JANUARY

Clasp Your Lover to Your Heart

The power of a soothing touch sometimes goes unappreciated in the West, even though everyone from infants to adults benefits from being touched and held. This lovely position, called the Clasping Position in the *Kama Sutra*, allows full-on, skin-to-skin body contact. You can do it with either partner on top, or even lying side-by-side.

After your partner is inside you, stretch your legs out and wrap them around his, still keeping them straight so that your feet touch. He then slides his hands underneath your shoulders and holds you to him while you do the same. This is a nice opportunity to tenderly stroke his shoulders, back, and bottom. While he may not be able to penetrate you very deeply, and your movements will be somewhat restricted, this position is deeply loving and intimate. Just keep undulating your hips so he won't think you've lost interest.

If you like, straighten your legs between his to tighten your vaginal opening and increase the friction on both his penis and your labia. He can even scoot up a bit so that his member rubs against your clitoris. Nice!

JANUARY

Treat Him to an Erotic Dance

And we don't mean a striptease. We'll save that for another day. What we're talking about here is the spontaneous, sexy dance of lust during coitus, where you move seemingly effortlessly from one position to another, following your own rhythm. After all, human beings express themselves not only through language but also through movement, and dancing is one of the most pleasurable forms of movement, as it allows us to convey a range of emotions and ideas. So if dancing can be sexy, why can't sex be like dancing? After all, people used to think that some forms of dancing encouraged fornication. Well, today we're going to let fornication encourage dancing—horizontal dancing, that is.

First, put on whatever music you'd use to seduce him on the dance floor. As you kiss and fondle each other, feel the music enter your blood as you become more and more excited. You might start making love missionary style, doing, say, the Clasping Position (see January 11). From there, you can move easily into the Twining Position, where you bend the knee of one leg and press your thigh against the back of his, weaving yourself around him and drawing him close. Do the same with the other leg and *voilà*! You're in the Pressing Position. From here, you can move your legs up, over and back down again as you bump and grind against him in time to the pulsing of the rhythm.

JANUARY

Position of the Week: Missionary Revisited

While it often gets maligned as boring or uninspired, there's a lot to be said for the good old Missionary position. It's comfortable during longer lovemaking sessions. It allows you to make eye contact and watch the passion on each other's faces throughout the deed. It lets you feel the wonderful sensations of skin against skin, heart against heart, and it makes deep, passionate kissing easy—a big plus if you're orally fixated.

Like most things in life, the Missionary is only as boring as the attitude you bring to it. After all, the wrong mindset can make the most acrobatic sexual pose ho-hum. Since this is a new month and a new year, let's approach the missionary with new enthusiasm and spend the next few days examining its variations.

Today, show how hot you are for him by guiding him inside you with your hands. As he begins to thrust inside you, match his every stroke with the movements of your hips. Grind against him. Rub your clitoris against his pubic bone. Swivel your hips as though you were belly dancing.

Now look deep into his eyes, and give him a few quick squeezes with your newly toned PC muscle. Clench him in time with his strokes. Vary the speed and rhythm of your squeezes until you're both over the moon.

JANUARY

Sex Queen (or King) for a Day!

In France, January 6 is *Le Jour des Rois* ("The Day of the Kings"), which the French celebrate by baking a small gift into the traditional *galette des rois*, or "cake of the kings." The person who finds the gift in their slice of cake is crowned king or queen for the evening.

Today, let's put a sexy twist on this Gallic tradition. Bake your absolutely favorite dessert cake, or if you're pressed for time, pick one up at your favorite bakery. The smaller the cake, the better. You'll see why in a minute! Before you put the cake in the oven, add a small charm to the batter, or carefully insert one into the finished dish. While the French often use tiny horseshoe shapes for luck, why not find something a little naughtier, like the key to a pair of furry handcuffs or a cock ring! Just make sure to wash it well before you add it to the cake.

Present the cake to your lover with a nice bottle of champagne, and announce that whoever finds the "lucky charm" gets to be Sex Queen (or King) for the night, with his or her every wish granted. This is guaranteed to make your sweetie's appetite return quickly, no matter how big a dinner you've just had.

What if no one finds the ring? There's always tomorrow night...

JANUARY

Sexual Fitness 1A

Around this time of year, the gyms are chock-full of people desperately trying to get their holiday-fattened bodies in shape. You, however, aren't going to the gym today, but you're still going to get fit. Sexually fit, that is. And the good news is that there's a single exercise that will do more to enhance your sex life than six months with Boris the Personal Trainer. It doesn't cost a cent, and you can do it anytime, anywhere. (The bad news? Actually, there is no bad news.) What is this magical erotic exercise? Strengthening your PC muscle.

The PC muscle (or pubococcygeus muscle, if you want to get technical) runs from your pubic bone to tailbone, surrounding your genitals. To find it, just stop the flow next time you pee: The muscle you use to do this is your PC. If you're not sure you're in the right place, slip a finger or two into your vagina and clench around them. Imagine gripping a lover's penis, and you'll get an idea of why it's called the "love muscle."

To strengthen your PC, simply squeeze the muscle and hold it for a few seconds. Then release. Do this a few more times. That's it! You've just learned to do *Kegel* exercises, named after the gynecologist who developed them. "Do your Kegels" a few times a day. Gradually, increase both your repetitions and the length of the contractions, and you'll be well on your way to sexual buffness.

JANUARY

Sexual Fitness 1B

How do I love my Kegel exercises? Let me count the ways.

Because it increases blood flow to the area, strengthening your PC enhances lovemaking whether you're alone or with a partner. A well-toned PC can increase clitoral sensations and vaginal lubrication, and produce more intense and stronger orgasms. Some claim it even helps achieve multiple orgasms. Men—who can do Kegels too—may enjoy easier, harder erections, and more control over their love shaft. What's not to like?

Yesterday, we learned a basic technique for exercising your love muscle. Today, let's try some slightly more advanced moves. First, synchronize your contractions with your breathing. When you squeeze your PC, inhale, and hold the contraction and your breath for a few seconds. Exhale and release. Just imagine you're in a sexual yoga class, because in a way, you are: Ancient Tantric texts extolled the virtues of a strong PC muscle.

You can also vary your speed. Clench quickly three to four times for each long squeeze, or bear down with your PC muscle, pressing out as though you were having a bowel movement, or giving birth. (Try to imagine something more romantic as you're doing this move.) These variations can be even more fun if you have something to clench around or push out—but that's tomorrow's tip.

There's no reason why you can't indulge your erotic imagination while doing your Kegels. Don a silk robe, recline languorously on some pillows, and imagine that you're a lady in ancient Japan preparing for the arrival of her lover. Now, isn't this better than step class?

JANUARY

The Position of Indrani

The *Kama Sutra* calls this next posture the Position of Indrani, after the wife of the Hindu king of the gods, Indra. What a saucy minx she must have been! As your man thrusts inside you, bend your knees up toward your ears, allowing him to penetrate your wet well deeply. If you can, press your calves against the backs of your thighs. You should be able to feel—and squeeze—against every inch of his shaft.

Because it allows such deep penetration, you may not want to stay in this position very long, but while you're here, make the most of it. Squeeze your butt muscles and rock your pelvis against him (like you were doing one of those lower abdominal crunches). The movement will be very small, but very subtle and delicious. From here, the choice is yours. Guide his hands to your breasts and nipples, or let him watch you caressing them yourself. Put your feet on his butt and pull him deeply inside you, or wrap your legs around his waist and grab his cheeks with your hands. Then rock with him to ecstasy!

HISTORICAL NOTE: Today is the birthday of Simone de Beauvoir (1908-86), French existentialist, writer, and essayist, whose ground-breaking book *The Second Sex* (1940) laid the groundwork for modern feminism.

JANUARY

Advanced Sexual Fitness (Don't Worry, It's Easy)

You can also speed up the PC toning process by adding resistance—that is, giving your love muscle something to squeeze around. This will help you gauge the strength of your flexing. Plus, it's fun.

Slide a clean finger, dildo, or vibrator into your vagina. In a pinch, you can use more organic objects like a carrot or cucumber. Just make sure you cover it with a condom, as we wouldn't want anything breaking off inside of you. Squeeze and hold for five to ten seconds. Relax and squeeze again, or do some quick squeezes (see January 4). Alternate by trying to push the finger or object out. Move the object around and enjoy the delicious sensations against your vaginal walls. Massage your clitoris, and see what lusty feelings it provokes. You can, of course, ask your lover to help you in this part of your erotic fitness regimen, but this may render concentration impossible.

If you love to shop, you can actually buy props to help you with your Kegels. If you have a sex-positive, woman-friendly store like Good Vibrations in your area, you'll probably be able to get devices such as the Kegelcisor there. The nice people there will be glad to help you. If you're not comfortable going into a store or are just pressed for time, go online. The Kegelcisor and other "pelvic muscle trainers" are even sold on mainstream sites like www.drugstore.com.

JANUARY

A Kiss Is More Than Just a Kiss

Whether it happens before, during or after, kissing can be one of the most intimate, erotic parts of lovemaking. As the saying goes, "As above, so below." The way someone kisses gives you a good idea of what kind of lover they'll be. Jane, a thirty-three-year-old financial planner, says, "Kissing is a critical part of foreplay. I love being kissed, and I love kissing my partner. It doesn't always have to be on the lips—I find the touch of his lips on any part of my body incredibly exciting."

Approach kissing like the sensual art it is. Before you even start, focus on your lover's lips and imagine how they'd feel on your skin. Then start out slow. Brush his lips with your ripe, voluptuous ones. Create a sense of anticipation. Give him a few gentle pecks first, as though you're deciding whether to go further. Savor the moment when your tongues first touch and begin to play with each other. Be creative by varying your speed, your pressure, and your urgency. Pull his lips gently between your teeth. Suck and nibble his mouth, especially his bottom lip. Pause, so that you can feel each other's breaths, then recommence your kisses with renewed ardor. Slide your tongue in and out of his mouth to show him what you'd like his penis to do to you later.

And don't forget how nice it can be to simply take your lover's face between your hands, showing him how much you cherish him, as you cover his mouth with kisses.

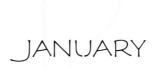

JANUARY

Give Him a Rest!

This posture is known as the Widely Opened Position in the *Kama Sutra*—maybe because the wider you open your legs, the more leverage you'll get. While he's on top of you in the missionary position, have him stop for a moment while you thrust and squeeze against him. Bend your knees, arch your back, and push up against him, bringing your hips off the mattress. (Think of it as a sexy version of yoga's Bridge Pose.) He may need to rise up on his knees a little bit as well—supporting himself on his arms—to give you room to maneuver. Let yourself go and throw your head back as you enjoy the delightful friction between your clitoris and his pubic bone.

The Refined Posture of the *Ananga Ranga* is very similar, except that your man kneels between your legs and pulls you up to him with his hands supporting your buttocks. If he draws your cheeks away from each other, he'll provide some extra erotic stimulation. Meanwhile, your hands are free to stroke his face, chest, and shoulders.

When you get tired or are just ready to move on, lower both your hips back to the mattress, and tilt your pelvis against him in slow, undulating motions. If you want to give him some exquisite torture, forbid him to move while you're doing this. See how long he can stand it.

JANUARY

Self-Loving Reason #1: Know Thyself (And Thy Sexual Response)

Each month, we're going to look at a different reason why masturbation is the key to sexual ecstasy. This month's reason is more than basic: Self-loving is the single best way—and perhaps the only way—for you to know what turns you on. If you don't know what gets you off, how do you expect your lover to? ESP? So get a grip on yourself—literally. Find out what kind of touch rocks your world. What kind of pressure and speed do you like—fast or slow? Hard or soft? Do you like stimulation throughout your orgasm, or does your clitoris become too sensitive once you've climaxed? Where's your G-spot, and what does it like? Can you have multiple orgasms? Only *you* can find the answers to these questions. Think of self-loving as a way to take inventory of your sexual assets so that you can exploit them to the fullest.

Masturbation teaches you how to play your most precious sexual instrument—your own body. And once you're an expert on playing solo, you'll be that much more ready for a beautiful duet.

JANUARY

Position of the Week: Splitting of a Bamboo

Since last week's position was the tried-and-true Missionary (although you can't say we didn't give you some fun variations), we'll start off this week with something a little bit more acrobatic from the *Kama Sutra*, a technique called The Splitting of a Bamboo. As your man enters you, raise your left leg onto his right shoulder and let it rest there as he thrusts inside you, leaving your right leg stretched out by his side. When you feel like it, lower your left leg and put your right leg on his left shoulder. Repeat as often as desired. The movement of your legs as you change positions—from which the position got its name—will cause your vagina to squeeze his penis and produce interesting sensations for both of you. Some people like the one-leg-over-the-shoulder position simply because it's such an interesting combination of brazen and coy.

A word about positions: As you've probably guessed by now, the *Kama Sutra* and most of the other ancient erotic texts describe activities that are just variations on the basics: Missionary, woman on top, side-by-side, rear entry, and sitting (or standing, which can be fun if you and your partner are the right heights). Sure, it can make you feel like a sexual superstar to use a clever name for some wacky arrangement of your limbs, but keep a sense of humor about it. It's more about finding inventive ways to enjoy and explore each other's bodies than following the instructions in a book.

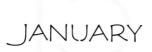

JANUARY

Express Yourself

This week, let's focus on another opening whose use as a sexual organ doesn't get enough attention—the mouth. And we're not just talking about its uses during oral sex, which we'll get to later. We're talking about *aural* sex. Good lovemaking makes use of all of our senses, including hearing. Most men find the sounds of passion incredibly erotic, so don't be afraid to express yourself during lovemaking. Your sighs, moans, and cries of ecstasy will make both of you hot.

Some people are shy about being vocal during an orgasm. Sometimes, having to be silent—like when you're visiting the in-laws and you don't want them to know what kind of vixen you are—can heighten the sense of daring and the intensity of your release, but if you hold back regularly, you're not experiencing the full pleasure of your climax. In fact, because you're repressing the heavy breathing of your natural orgasmic response, your silence may actually stifle the power of your orgasm. So let 'er rip. Not only will you enjoy your orgasm more, but so will your lover.

Equally important is that you listen to the sounds you and your lover make while you're together. His moans will help you respond to his moves and desires. It's hard to make beautiful music with a silent partner.

JANUARY

Midnight Striptease Surprise

When it's cold outside, who could blame you for cozying up in your warmest flannel PJs? Certainly not your guy. But tonight, give him a sexy surprise. Wait until he's fast asleep, and then doff the flannels in favor of your birthday suit. Imagine how excited he'll be when he rolls over to cuddle with you in the morning—or the middle of the night—and puts his arms around your satiny-soft skin instead of fabric. You can even hurry things along by guiding his sleepy hands to your bare breast, the curve of your derriere, or the warm wetness between your legs. Better yet, slide under the covers and wake him up with your warm mouth on his member. He may think he's dreaming!

JANUARY

Share a Fantasy

There's no reason to be ashamed of fantasizing, whether you're alone or with a partner. In fact, a Kinsey survey found that more than seventy percent of men and women have fantasized during sex with a partner. You've probably heard the saying that "ninety-nine percent of sex occurs between the ears," reminding us that when it comes to sex organs, the brain is the largest.

Since this is a month of openings and beginnings, start by being open with your partner by sharing one of your sexual fantasies. If you're new to each other, start with one of your tamer ones and see what the reaction is. It can be an incredible turn-on for a partner to know your mind harbors such lusty thoughts.

And since turn about is fair play, ask your partner to tell you one of his fantasies. (Don't be shocked by whatever it is. That wouldn't be playing fair.) Simply talking about and describing your secret sexual thoughts with each other can act as an incredible aphrodisiac and, because it's such a revealing, intimate act, bring you closer together— which makes for even hotter sex.

Take note that it doesn't mean you have to act your fantasies out— unless you want to. One way to do this safely is by having your partner talk through your fantasy next time you're making love or masturbating for each other. You'll both be aroused in no time.

JANUARY

1-800-LUST

People sometimes talk about phone sex as though it's evil, but in truth, they're missing out. If you're separated from your sweetie—even if it's only for a day—phone sex can be a safe, fun way to keep your sexual engine purring. And as an instrument of seduction, the phone has few equals. If you haven't done the deed yet, letting your partner hear what you sound like in the throes of passion will put his erotic imagination into overdrive.

Say your partner's on a business trip. Set up a time to talk that night, and prepare yourself just as though you were going to sleep with him. Take a warm, steamy bath, rub your body with oil, put on your sexiest lingerie, and slip between the sheets. Perhaps even light some candles. Here's the most important part: When you pick up the phone, *turn off call waiting*. Nothing is going to kill the mood faster than Mom ringing through to chat just as you're approaching the Big O.

The secret to great phone sex is describing everything. And that means *everything*. Let him hear you touching your erect nipples, your smooth belly, your bodacious booty, your moist slit. Let him hear your gasps of delight as you rub your love button. Ask him to tell you what he'd be doing to you if he were there. When you come, don't hold back. He'll be counting the minutes until the next time he sees you.

JANUARY

The Yawning Position

In the *Kama Sutra*, the following position is called the Yawning Position, but it's unlikely you'll fall asleep while doing it. While in the missionary position, raise your legs and part them widely. Change the angle of your thighs to increase or decrease how deeply he penetrates you, or experiment with slipping a pillow under your hips. Your lover can also rise up onto his knees and lean forward to press against your thighs and support them. While this position may not afford much clitoral stimulation—a situation either one of you can fix with creative use of your hands—it does give the man a great view of his slick member sliding in and out of the petals of your lovely vulva. It also encourages a feeling of delicious erotic abandon as you open yourself wide to him.

If you're limber, you can vary the Yawning Position by lifting your legs even higher and placing one foot on either side of his head while you rest your calves on his shoulders. He can caress your legs and feet or hold them to steady himself. For a deliciously lustful sensation for both of you, squeeze your thighs tightly around his member.

Because he'll be able to penetrate you even more deeply, you'll want to be fully aroused before you try this move. You may even feel him bumping against your cervix. Some women find this highly pleasurable. If you don't, you'll want to let him know so he can ease off on his thrusts, or so you can change your position altogether.

JANUARY

Full Body Kissing

Here's a game to warm you up on a cold winter's night. Tell your lover that you're going to shower his naked body with kisses. Start at the top of his head and work your way down. Run your tongue along the inside of his ears. Nuzzle his neck. Tease his nipples. Trace the outline of his ribs with your mouth. Drag your tongue lightly across his abs and brush your lips along the inside of his thighs. Your mouth shouldn't leave an inch of his skin untouched. Turn him over and do the same to his shoulders, back, buttocks, and backs of his legs. Explore every nook and cranny of his body, but leave his privates alone for now.

Here's the most important part: As you explore each body part with your mouth, he has to tell you how much he likes it on a scale of one to ten. Then switch roles, and have him do the same to you.

What's the point of all this oral teasing, other than a way to stave off cabin fever? First, it creates an incredible sense of erotic anticipation. Second, it's a fabulous way to get to know each other's pleasure spots—other than the genitals. Remember that saying about the brain as a sexual organ? Well, the skin is another one. Don't neglect it, especially during those times of the year when you spend most of your time covering it up.

HISTORICAL NOTE: Today is the birthday of Federico Fellini (1920-1993), Italian director of films such as *La Dolce Vita* (1960), *Fellini's Casanova* (1976), and *Fellini Satyricon* (1969), which portrayed debauchery in Rome under Nero's rule.

JANUARY

The Age of Aquarius

If you or your lover were born between this date and February 19, you fall under the sign of Aquarius, the water bearer. Aquarians are known for their independent, freewheeling personalities, and their individualistic nature, which makes them fascinating friends and lovers. If you're in love with an Aquarian, be prepared to go with the flow. Seduce your Aquarian honey by appealing to his love of spontaneity. Suggest an *al fresco* romp or point out an unusual position in the *Kama Sutra*. The more unconventional, the better.

If you are an Aquarian yourself—or simply want to experience the Aquarian mindset—*you* initiate the quickie. Be impetuous. Let him know that you have to have him right *now*. Grab his package, bend over the dining room table, and offer him your bewitching behind. Don't feel guilty about being late to dinner or whatever (not that you would). A quickie is a great way to release tension, boost endorphins, and improve your mood. Best of all, everyone will wonder why the two of you are wearing such big smiles all evening.

JANUARY

Position of the Week: Southern Cross

Here's a position that sounds complicated, but really isn't. Lie on your back, with your right leg straight out and your left leg at a ninety-degree angle, bent at the knee. He lies on his right side facing and perpendicular to you, so that your bodies form a cross. Lift your left leg and drape it over his hip as he enters you (at the center of the cross); your right leg will slide between his.

The nice thing about this position is that it's comfortable, especially if you've been making love for a while, and it offers unimpeded access to your clitoris, which either of you can pleasure with your hands or a vibrator as he thrusts inside you. You can also gaze into each other's eyes throughout the act.

HISTORICAL NOTE: Lord Byron (1788-1824), the leading poet of the Romantic movement, was born today. After fleeing England to escape a failed marriage and rumors of an incestuous relationship with his half-sister, he lived a life worthy of one of his own epic poems, dying while helping the Greeks fight for their independence.

JANUARY

Oral Sex—Her Turn, Slowly

It's time for one of his openings to make contact with yours: his mouth, your vagina (and its nearby attractions). Some women are shy about letting a man go down on them. Don't be. A survey in *Cosmopolitan* found that seventy percent of men love performing oral sex on their woman. And as long as you keep yourself clean, most guys like your natural smell, so for God's sake, don't douche. The vagina is designed to be a self-cleaning organ, and douches disturb its natural pH balance. So leave the chemicals out of the playground.

We'll be covering oral sex for both parties throughout the year, but today, let's keep it simple. No matter how exotic the tricks, the secret to great cunnilingus is *communication*. Tell him what you like. If you don't know, now's the time for you to find out together. So just for today, ask him to go slow. Tell him you'd like it if he explored your entire garden of love with his mouth instead of heading straight to your clit. Ask him to work from the outside in, from your inner thighs to the inside of your furry labia majora to your petal-like inner lips, before he finally reaches your love button. Suggest that he caress your entire vulva in long strokes. As you revel in the sensations of his insistent tongue, run your fingers through his hair, and let him hear your cries of delight.

HISTORICAL NOTE: John Cleland, author of *Fanny Hill: or the Memoirs of a Woman of Pleasure,* was born today in 1709 in London. The book, considered the first "erotic novel," was subsequently banned in both England and the United States until 1966, when the U.S. Supreme Court ruled that it did not meet the Roth standard for obscenity.

JANUARY

Oral Sex—His Turn, Slowly

If you want to be an expert at giving your man oral pleasure, take a cue from yesterday's tip and *go slow*. Take your time. Just like you wouldn't want him to go straight for your clitoris while ignoring all the other nearby attractions, don't go straight for the head of his penis. Most of the nerve endings are located there, so it's much too sensitive for a full-on attack right from the get-go. (Think popsicle, not lollipop, until he gets warmed up.) Instead, let his anticipation build. Start out by gazing at and stroking his rock-hard erection. Shower it with kisses. If he's not hard yet, simply draw his entire penis into your mouth and gently suck and lick; wait until he's partially erect before you start moving up and down. Making a ring around the base with your thumb and forefinger will make him hard faster.

When he's ready, kiss the glans and wet it with your tongue. Run the tip of your tongue along the supersensitive ridge between the head and the shaft. Then, keep your lips over your teeth and slowly slide his waiting member into your mouth, and then down as far as you can go. Apply the strongest pressure to the bottom of his shaft as you move your head up and down in smooth, continuous movements. At this point, the key to sending your man over the edge is rhythm. Try to keep up a constant pace, gradually increasing your speed as he writhes in ecstasy. Enjoy the pleasure you're giving him—he is!

JANUARY

Take Notes!

Use the power of the written word to send your man into paroxysms of erotic anticipation. Leave him sexy notes where he's sure to find them: In his pants or coat pocket, taped to the bathroom mirror, or resting on his computer keyboard. Liven up his boring staff meeting by sending him a naughty text message. When he travels, slip a racy note into his suitcase. Ideally, he'll get the message (literally) and pay you back in kind.

Karen, a thirtysomething lawyer who travels frequently on business, recounts how her boyfriend puts notes in her suitcase with messages like "I think you're beautiful and can't wait for you to come home," "Call me so I can tell you what I'd like to be doing to your body," or simply "I miss you." Her favorite note, she says, was a domestic "I'll do the laundry and vacuum before you get home."

Karen also says that her lusty man occasionally throws a naked snapshot of himself into her luggage. Assuming you trust your dude, try this yourself. Learn how to use your camera's self-timer or ask a trusted friend to help you with a boudoir shot. Or innocently ask him to take pictures of you with your own camera, and surprise him with them later. After all, men—God bless 'em—are visual creatures. Use this to your advantage! And remember that a picture always speaks louder than words.

JANUARY

Oral Sex and the Love Button

Here's a tip designed for sharing with your partner. You can either describe it or show him this page. After he's warmed up the rest of your vulva, ask him to focus on your clitoris. Don't put any pressure on yourself to climax. If you do, great, but this is his chance to explore the landscape, and your chance to find out more about what turns you on. Ask him to caress each side of your clitoris and circle it with his tongue. He can even take the entire clitoris in his mouth and kiss it deeply. You can experiment with whether you like to have your love button sucked or nibbled lightly. For some women, this is too much stimulation, while it sends others through the roof.

As your clit becomes harder and you get more aroused, pay attention to the sensations. Do you want him to go faster? Slower? Harder? Softer? Or keep up a constant, steady pressure (which most women prefer)? Does one side feel better than the other? Let him know. Hopefully, he'll be taking note of your moaning, deep breathing, and rocking hips, but it never hurts to drive the point home; be specific, or say something along the lines of "Oh my God! Right there! Just like that!" When it comes to the clitoris, clarity counts.

HISTORICAL NOTE: Today is the birthday of Eartha Kitt (1928-), American actress and singer known for her "sex kitten" style.

JANUARY

Tongue and Finger

Another nice technique to try while your partner goes down on you is to ask him to slip a finger inside your wet vagina. The sensation of being penetrated during oral sex drives many women wild. For variation, have him replace his finger with a buzzing vibrator or your favorite dildo.

Play with whatever turns you on the most, such as a finger just at your moist entrance, barely inserted, perhaps up the knuckle; or even two fingers. If it doesn't distract you, he can slide it slowly in and out, mimicking the action of his erect penis. You might prefer that he just hold it still, so you can enjoy the feeling of being penetrated as he teases your clitoris into ecstasy. Or he can crook his finger, as though he were beckoning you closer, and press against your G-spot. Relax and surrender to the incredible feelings coursing through your body.

JANUARY

Position of the Week: 69

Going down on each other at the same time allows you to explore each other's lower openings with your mouth and fingers. Some people may find that they have trouble concentrating on their own pleasure in this position. If that's the case for you, don't worry about having an orgasm—just enjoy your lover's mouth on you while you're merrily sucking away at his love shaft. (You won't be able to slide your mouth up and down his member much unless you're the one on top.)

A few tips for getting the most from this position: If your man's on top, experiment with how high his hips need to be above your head. If he's lying flat on you, he may penetrate your mouth too deeply; if he's too high up on his knees, his penis may not reach you at all, and you don't want to strain your neck bobbing for it. It's okay to gently guide his hips up or down until you're both comfortable. Of course, if you're on top, you can easily control the pressure of your clit on his tongue as you practice your oral skills on his grateful member.

If either of you come in this position, great! Or you may simply want to use it as a warm-up for your main course.

HISTORICAL NOTE: Colette (Sidonie Gabrielle Claudine Colette, 1873-1954), the French novelist whose work explored human relationships, especially physical relationships, was born today in the village of Saint-Saveur-en-Puisaye, Burgundy, France.

JANUARY

Discover Your Back Door

Since this is the month of openings, let's forget an oft-neglected orifice—your anus. Don't leave it out of your erotic repertoire, or you'll be missing out. Your nerve-rich anal tissues get engorged, tense up, and contract when you get turned on, just like your other sexual organs. To some people, anal play's taboo nature makes it even more of a turn-on.

Start by exploring the area on your own. If you just take a little extra time to clean back there with a damp cloth, baby wipe or soapy finger, you'll be fine—feces only hang out in the rectum right before you use the bathroom—and a freshly cleaned bum greatly reduces the squeamish factor.

Get comfortable, and wet your index or middle finger with a good water-based lubricant. Because the anus doesn't produce its own lubrication, you should *always* have lube on hand any time you indulge in anal pleasure. Saliva and vaginal juices aren't going to be enough. Begin by massaging lovingly around the opening, including the sensitive *perineum*, the spot between your vulva and anus. Relax and breathe. Slowly and gently, slide one fingertip inside. Proceed further as you feel comfortable. Try tightening your sphincter muscles around your finger. Experiment with circular motions and different levels of pressure. Angle your finger forward, and see how it feels against your G-spot. (Just remember: *Never* put anything that's been in your anus into your vagina.) Take pleasure in the lovely new sensual feelings—and erotic possibilities—that anal play delivers.

HISTORICAL NOTE: Today is the birthday of Germaine Greer (1939-), Australian writer and feminist, and author of *The Female Eunuch.*

JANUARY

Discover His Back Door

Many straight men are missing out on an incredibly erotic experience simply because they think that enjoying anal eroticism means they're homosexual. Silly boys. It's who you make love to—not how—that determines your sexual orientation. So if you've got an open-minded or experimental lover, don't ignore this exquisitely sensitive part of his body. If you're at all squeamish, take a bath or shower together and clean every inch of each other first.

The keys to enjoyable anal play are communication, relaxation, and lots and lots of lubrication. Make sure he knows what you're intending to do. Maybe he just wants you to circle a well-lubed finger around his opening. That's fine. Take your time. Encourage him to breathe and relax; eventually, he may be able to bear down on your finger, or you can slowly slip a fingertip into him. Point toward his belly button rather than his back as you slide in up to the knuckle, and wait for his anus and sphincter muscles to accustom themselves. Slowly circle or stroke the rectum walls at a slow pace. Combine this with oral sex or manual stimulation, and you'll drive him wild.

SAFE SEX NOTE: Engage in anal play only if you're sure of your partner's sexual health. To be really safe, use a lubricated latex glove or finger cot. This has the added bonuses of alleviating any hygiene issues and protecting delicate tissues from your fingernails—even though you'll have clipped them before you start playing with his bum, right?

JANUARY

*"If I had to live my life again,
I'd make the same mistakes, only sooner."*
—Tallulah Bankhead

Your Openings, Two at a Time

Let's take some time to get creative. You can enjoy some amazingly sensual sensations by slipping one finger inside your vulva and another well-lubricated finger into your anus, and rubbing against the delicate internal wall between the vaginal and anal canals. To do this, spread your legs and slip a hand under your luscious behind. Experiment with using one hand, leaving your thumb or other hand free to massage your clitoris or your hardening nipples. Or slide your thumb inside your vagina and your middle finger in your anus, and gently clasp the two together as you stroke your clitoris with abandon. If it's too awkward for either or both hands, try using your favorite vibrator or dildo in either opening. (You don't use a vibrator? We'll get to that.)

Indulge in naughty fantasies of being penetrated by two lusty lovers at once as you bring yourself to ecstasy. Just imagine how excited your own lover will be when you show him how you've started off the New Year!

HISTORICAL NOTE: Actress Tallulah Bankhead was born today in 1902 in Huntsville, Alabama. Outrageous and uninhibited, Bankhead appeared in almost every medium—stage, film, radio, and television—but was also known for her wild antics and numerous affairs.

CHAPTER TWO

FEBRUARY

"Late February days; and now, at last,
Might you have thought that Winter's woe was past;
So fair the sky was and so soft the air."
—*William Morris,* The Earthly Paradise

February takes its name from the Latin word *februa*, after the festivals of purification celebrated in ancient Rome around this time of year. This February, we'll talk about ways to create your own sensual purification rituals, from soothing, sexy baths to candlelit lovemaking sessions incorporating Tantric breathing techniques.

The Victorians assigned several meanings to this month's birth flower, the beautiful *primrose*, from "I can't live without you" to "early youth" or "young love." Fill a vase with primroses to symbolize that this month, you'll approach your sexuality with the excitement, passion, and creativity of a young lover, delighting in her lover's body as a playground of new sensual delights.

Find a way to incorporate the rich purple color of February's birthstone, *amethyst*, into your surroundings to remind yourself of what it symbolizes: sincerity. This February, you'll be sincerely true to your desires!

FEBRUARY

Take a Bath Together!

Since ancient times, baths have been used not only for personal hygiene and relaxation but also as part of religious purification rituals and as opportunities for social interaction. Tonight, create your own sensual purification ritual with your lover by taking a bath together! Set the mood by lighting candles and playing soft music. Adjust the water temperature to suit your desires (a hot bath is stimulating, while skin-temperature water has a relaxing effect). Don't forget the bubble bath and a couple of inflatable neck pillows.

Once you're both soaking, have fun getting each other squeaky clean. Sit between his legs, and ask him to scrub your back with a loofah. Lie back against his chest, and let him play with your soapy nipples, gently clean the folds of your labia, and caress between your buttocks with a warm washcloth. Allow yourself to feel pampered and indolent. When it's his turn, have him turn around so you can massage his back, then face you as you work your way down his body. Order him to hold still as you lovingly administer to his penis, scrotum, and even lower. If your heart's not already racing with lust, a hot bath will quicken your pulse and breathing. You may find yourselves adjourning to the bedroom before too long!

If you don't have a bathtub, see if your health club or spa has private hot tub rooms. In the San Francisco Bay Area, for example, there's a wonderful place called Watercourse Way (www.watercourseway.com) that offers beautiful rooms, some with steam rooms and cold plunges, but all with day beds for resting after your dip. With any luck, you won't feel like resting!

FEBRUARY

Wet 'n Wild

Flying solo tonight? You can have a lot of fun in the tub by yourself—
a *lot* of fun. Turn on the water in the bathtub, and lie on your back in
the tub, using a bath pillow to cushion your neck, shoulders, and head.
Slide your derriere as close as possible to the wall near the faucet, open
your hips, and extend your legs up the wall. Adjust your body so that
your back doesn't hurt, and tilt your clitoris up toward the stream of
water. If you're very limber, adjust the water pressure and temperature
with your toes; if you're less coordinated, you may have to reach up a
few times to get everything right. See what happens when you spread
your inner lips. As the water pelts your privates, enjoy the sensations,
which some women describe as getting a good licking!

Don't have a bathtub? Invest in a faucet attachment that has a handheld showerhead on a hose. The versatile showerhead offers you lots of
different settings, from a strong, steady jet to a pulsating stream. Just
be sure you don't get carried away and slip!

HISTORICAL NOTE: Havelock Ellis (1859-1939), the pioneering
British psychologist, was born today. Ellis was the author of the ground-
breaking, seven-volume *Studies in the Psychology of Sex*, which was
banned for several years and only available to the medical profession
until 1935. A supporter of women's rights, sexual liberation, and birth
control, Ellis and his work greatly influenced the scientific study of sex.

FEBRUARY

Meet Your G-Spot

In this month of purification, let's purify our minds about the infamous G-spot. More mystery surrounds this alleged hot button than the last appearance of Bigfoot. Does it really exist? Where is it? How do I find it? Relax. Every woman has a G-spot: It's actually the urethral sponge, the tissue that surrounds your urethra and runs along the front of your vaginal wall for about one or two inches. It's called the "G-spot"—even though it's not really a spot so much as an area—after Ernest Gräfenberg, the gynecologist who first wrote about it in 1950.

Here's how to learn what delights your own G-spot provides. Remember, each woman's response to G-spot stimulation will vary. Some women claim it gives them stupendous orgasms, while others find it leaves them cold. However, do spend a little time pleasuring yourself before you go hunting—your G-spot will be easier to find if you're aroused. When you're ready, slip a lubricated finger inside your vagina. By crooking your finger along the front wall of your vagina, you should find a ridged spongy area (right behind the pubic bone) that feels different from the smooth vaginal walls. Press firmly, as the G-spot can only be felt *through* the vaginal wall.

Now you're free to find out what pressure your sweet spot likes. Try massaging it by moving your finger side-to-side, or by stroking it in a circle. Experiment with different positions: lying down, sitting, squatting, or lying on your stomach. See what happens if you press down on your abdomen at the same time. Continue to stimulate yourself to find out what raptures result. If nothing happens, don't sweat it. Find something else you like!

HISTORICAL NOTE: Gertrude Stein (1874-1946), the avant-garde American writer whose Paris salon attracted artists and writers including Pablo Picasso and Ernest Hemingway, was born today. Stein lived openly with her lifelong companion, Alice B. Toklas.

FEBRUARY

Position of the Week: Rear Entry

There's a lot to be said for doing it "Doggie Style." It lets him penetrate you deeply, and he's more likely to hit your G-spot. He can play with your nipples and clitoris, and it gives him a great view of your fine booty. And heck, isn't there something just a little bit primal about hearing his thighs slap against you? If the thought of all this makes you feel a little too nasty, you can comfort yourself with the thought that rear entry is the Sixth Posture of *The Perfumed Garden*, the sixteenth-century Arabian text by Sheikh Nefzawi. It also appears in the Taoist sex manual *T'ung Hsüan Tzu* as The White Tiger position.

Best of all, this position is easy. Just get on your hands and knees, supporting yourself on your elbows if you need to. Spread your thighs slightly, angle your buttocks, and present your lovely, wet vagina to your partner as he enters you from behind. Push back to meet his thrusts, and tilt your pelvis so that every inch of your vulva touches him when you collide. Although he can caress your back and derriere and grasp your hips as he pounds into you, encourage him to stroke your nipples and engorged clitoris until you both lose yourself in erotic frenzy.

HISTORICAL NOTE: Today is the birthday of feminist leader Betty Friedan (1921-), founder of the National Organization of Women (NOW), and author of *The Feminine Mystique*, which challenged long-held assumptions about women's roles.

FEBRUARY

Self-Loving Reason #2: Reconnect with Your Body

Self-pleasuring isn't just a way to become more familiar with your sexual response—it's also a great way to reconnect with your body. In today's fast-paced world, most of us spend way too much time in our heads. We sit at computers all day and plop in front of the television at night. We numb-out with food, drugs, alcohol, and even sex. We eat when we're not hungry. We stay up even though we're tired. Even when we exercise, we work out to the television, radio, music—anything so that we're not alone with our thoughts and our bodies. And guess what? Our body sends us reliable, insistent bulletins that we're ignoring it. We get stress headaches. Stomach problems. Injuries. Libido issues.

Masturbation can put us right back in touch with the sensations and desires of our neglected bodies. Next time you're playing with yourself, note how each part of your body responds, starting from the top of your head. Does your face feel warm? How does your skin feel? Your breasts and nipples? Do your stomach muscles tighten? How are you breathing? What exactly happens at the moment you achieve an orgasm? If you can stay present with yourself, you'll be able to stay present with a lover—and that will make sex explosively intimate for both of you.

HISTORICAL NOTE: Today is the birthday of Charlotte Rampling (1945-), the British actress known for her sensual and daring roles in movies like *The Night Porter* (1973) and the recent *Swimming Pool* (2003).

FEBRUARY

Set the Stage

For the next few days, we're going to focus on your surroundings, starting with your bedroom. A well-designed space can affect your mood and possibly even your health. You wouldn't want to eat a gourmet meal in a dingy, messy storage locker; why would you want to make love there? Take some time to create a space that's a shrine to spectacular sex.

You don't have to spend a lot of money to have a sensuous boudoir. If you do nothing else, keep your bedroom as clutter-free as possible. Clutter is distracting and anxiety-provoking—two emotions at odds with arousal. You don't want to be tripping over last week's laundry on your way to the bed. The only thing that should be on the floor is your underwear—after he rips it off you. Likewise, clear off the furniture. How is he going to lift your sweet butt up on to the dresser for some sexy standing schtupping if it's covered with jewelry, makeup, and knick-knacks?

Clearing out clutter can be a freeing activity. As you get rid of all the junk that no longer serves you, you'll feel lighter, more relaxed, and sexier. When you're done, light a candle or some incense. Create your own personal ritual to honor the fact that you've just made room for new love and new pleasure.

FEBRUARY

The Bounteous Bed

The center stage of your bedroom is, of course, your bed, and at the minimum you should invest in a queen-sized mattress. A twin or a double is only exciting if you're trying to sneak some nooky in your parents' guest room, or if you're a college student. Otherwise, a small bed makes engaging in amatory gymnastics impossible. As far as your mattress goes, the type is up to you, although it should be firm and comfortable. And make sure you have a sturdy boxspring and bed frame. You don't want to crash to the floor in the middle of the action.

The best kind of bed is one that makes you want to dive into it and roll around. Think *sensuous*. Clean sheets, preferably cotton, are a must. Buy the highest thread count you can afford, and you'll be rewarded with luxurious softness against your bare skin night after night. Pillows come in handy, so try to invest in more than one. You can lounge back against them like an indolent harem girl or stick one under your hips to give him better access to your private parts. Please try to avoid scratchy bedspreads or frilliness of any kind, and whatever you do, no stuffed animals, unless that really, really turns you (or him) on.

To headboard or not to headboard? Again, up to you, but it might be best to avoid a solid footboard: you want to make it "access easy" from any angle and ensure that there's enough space for feet and arms to dangle off the bed. So go without, unless you like something to which you could tie a silk scarf or velvet cuffs, you naughty minx.

FEBRUARY

What's on Your Nightstand?

While a certain fashion magazine likes asking celebrities what books are on their nightstands, if you want to set the stage for seduction, stow your reading material somewhere else—unless it's a book of erotica and you're planning to read him some "bedtime stories." Otherwise, the two of you will feel like you're in a library. Besides, looking at all those unread books will only make you feel guilty.

What your nightstand *should* hold is everything you need for great sex. Ideally, it will have a small drawer in which you can stow condoms, sex toys, massage oils, and lubricant. Be sure that the condoms, especially, are within easy reach. You don't want to have to go digging through your nightstand drawer when you'd rather be digging through *his* drawers.

While some suggest keeping a box of tissues by the bed, you may want to consider these words of advice from *Sex Tips for Straight Women from a Gay Man* by Dan Anderson and Maggie Berman: "Semen is sticky, and let's face it, a guy feels pretty ridiculous having tissues stuck to his penis after sex." Stow a clean washcloth or towel in your nightstand instead, or, as they suggest, keep a pump bottle of unscented body lotion by the bed for massages and manual play—and for keeping your skin baby soft, of course.

HISTORICAL NOTE: Today is the birthday of Lana Turner (1920-95), the American film actress known as MGM's "Sweater Girl."

FEBRUARY

The Eyes Have It

Besides having a good bed, no clutter, and a well-equipped nightstand, what else can you do to make your bedroom a haven for sensuality? Think about appealing to all of your five senses. Most men are visually oriented, so let's start there.

First, make sure that there's enough light for him to see you and the erotic acts you're doing together. The lighting in your bedroom, including your bedside lamp, shouldn't be too bright: You don't want to feel like you're undergoing an interrogation (unless that's one of your fantasies). A lamp with a dimmer switch is perfect, and while candles are sexy, put them where you won't have to worry that the bed linens are going to catch fire while you're rolling about. Finally, a mirror can be a nice touch. A full-length antique mirror or mirrored closet doors let you both enjoy watching the action.

It goes without saying that you should be careful what photos are on display. Nothing can kill the mood faster than looking up during the throes of passion and seeing a photo of your ex, or say, Grandma. However, if you're married or in a relationship, you can put a photo of the two of you in what feng shui experts call the relationship corner, which is usually the southwest corner of the room. If you're single, put a picture of yourself in this corner. This isn't narcissistic. To be a good lover, you first have to have self-confidence, and you do that by cultivating the most important relationship of all: with yourself.

FEBRUARY

Victorian Erotica

Looking for some inspiration to get those sexual fires burning? Erotic literature—erotica—can now be found in most bookstores. During Victorian times, however, erotic classics like *The Pearl* (now available on audiocassette!) and *My Secret Life* circulated underground to great acclaim. *The Pearl*, a magazine that published erotic short stories, verse, and serialized novels, first appeared in London in July 1887 and lasted for eighteen months before vanishing, its publishers unable to make ends meet. While it may not win any awards for literary genius—and it certainly can't be accused of political correctness—the erotica found in *The Pearl* is explicit, kinky, and undeniably hot.

The nice thing about erotica, especially classic erotica, is that it lets us safely explore situations and practices that we might never try in real life. My friend Alex, a happily married, twentysomething graduate student, keeps a secret stash of Victorian erotica that she reads while pleasuring herself. "I particularly like stories about orgies, although I have to admit that the *idea* of participating in one is more exciting to me than the prospect of actually participating in one," she says. Like any good book, good erotica lets us enjoy a variety of sexual experiences without the mess and fuss, the inconvenient smells, and the emotional minefields of real life. On this cold February night, curl up with a good dirty book from a bygone era, and see where it takes you.

FEBRUARY

Position of the Week: Rear Entry, Lying Down

A very sweet variation on Doggie Style is to do it lying down. You lie flat on your stomach as he lies on top of you, slipping his penis between your buttocks and slightly parted legs to enter you. If he arches his back and supports himself on his hands and forearms, he'll be able to penetrate you more deeply. A pillow under your hips will also make your inviting vulva more accessible, and keep him from slipping out. Encourage him to kiss and nuzzle your shoulders and the back of your neck. Take his hands in yours—maybe even bestow a few kisses on his palm or suck one of his fingers—to deepen the erotic charge between you. To make thrusting easier, he can grip his toes on the edge of the bed or hold your shoulders.

While you may enjoy very intense G-spot stimulation from this position, the only drawback is that it may be hard for either of you to fondle your clitoris. You can get around this easily by placing a vibrator under you. Imagine the sensations as he thrusts into you!

In ancient, sacred erotic texts, this position has several different names, from the Elephant Posture in the *Kama Sutra* to the *T'ung Hsüan Tzu's* lovely Cicada on a Bough. *The Perfumed Garden* simply calls it Coitus from the Back, terming it "the easiest of all methods." Only if you're really tired!

HISTORICAL NOTE: Today is the birthday of Virginia Eshelman Johnson (1925-), the American researcher who teamed with William Masters to measure human sexual behavior, which resulted in the groundbreaking book *Human Sexual Response* (1966).

FEBRUARY

Seduce Yourself

On a cold winter's night, a little self-seduction can really stoke your fires. But don't just flop on the bed and stick your hand between your legs. Put the moves on yourself. If you're lucky enough to have a fireplace, build a blazing fire and stretch out on a soft blanket and a bunch of pillows. Or put your best sheets on the bed and light some candles. Turn off the phone, and put on your favorite mood music. Take a nice, hot bath, and drink a glass of wine or a steaming cup of tea. Thumb through your favorite collection of erotica. Do whatever you need to do to get yourself in the mood.

But don't forget the foreplay. Massage your breasts. Tease your nipples. Rub your hands over your belly, down between your legs. Massage your mons pubis and the outside of your vulva. Wet your fingers on your own sweet juices, then gradually move up to your delicate rosebud. Once you arrive at your now-erect nub, use whatever method you prefer to bring yourself to ecstasy. You've got a whole year to experiment with different techniques!

If you haven't experienced an orgasm yet, don't chase it. Let it come to you. Take time to get to know your body. Remember, today's tip is to seduce yourself. Pressure and seduction are mutually exclusive. Tonight is all about you, at your pace.

FEBRUARY

Use Your Scents

Don't overlook your sense of smell as you create your erotic love nest. Smells can exert a powerful sensory effect over us—even an erotic one. In fact, a 1998 study by the Smell & Taste Treatment and Research Foundation found that the combined scent of lavender and pumpkin pie increased penile blood flow by forty percent!

Whether they're in your house or on your person, use scents in moderation. Anoint yourself with a dab of your signature perfume or cologne on the pulse points at your wrists, neck, and even behind your kneecaps. Your body chemistry will interact with the fragrance to make it your own, and remind your lover of you even when you're not there. (I can't walk past my man's closet without thinking of him, because his clothes are imbued with the wonderful masculine cologne he uses.) You want your lover to associate your scent with sensuality, not sneezing. Same goes for scented candles, incense and the like. A whiff is plenty.

But when it comes to perfume, your lover may find the scent of your freshly washed body to be the most enticing. Don't forget the power of pheromones. Research has shown that these airborne chemical signals even influence humans. Why would you want to cover up the tools nature gave you to help attract a mate? Sure, you may not want to get it on right after a two-hour kickboxing class, but who knows? Sometimes there's nothing as good as hot, sweaty, lusty sex. Next time you're making love, close your eyes and concentrate on the sweet erotic bouquet produced by your passion.

FEBRUARY

My Erotic Valentine

Find your own way to celebrate love this Valentine's Day, whether it's by doing something special for your lover, your loved ones, or yourself. Here's one idea for having your own X-rated celebration at home.

First, turn your living room into an erotic playspace. Move the coffee table to one side and push back the couches. Build a fire in the fireplace or light a bunch of candles. Spread out a soft blanket or comforter, and set up lots of pillows and cushions. Cook a romantic meal—"romantic" meaning anything delicious and easy to prepare—with or without a partner. Spread out your meal on a blanket, and take turns feeding each other. Have lots of your favorite beverage on hand. You can decide what to wear, whether it's your sexiest outfit or nothing at all. (You get extra bonus points for shaving or waxing your pubic hair into a heart shape.)

Now for the evening's main attraction. Take ten to fifteen minutes to write as many "sexual favors" as you can both think of on slips of paper. These favors are anything you would love for your partner to do to or for you. (Play fair: Don't list activities to which you know he or she would object.) Fold up the slips and put them in separate bowls, and take turns drawing "favors" from each other's bowls. The anticipation will drive you both crazy, and you'll have fun granting each other's favorite sensual desires.

There's no reason at all you can't create an erotic atmosphere if you happen to be alone—simply use the evening as an excuse to indulge yourself by doing whatever it is you *love* to do, whether it's watching your favorite movie, eating your favorite foods, losing yourself in a novel, or pleasuring yourself!

FEBRUARY

Lupercalia

In ancient Rome, today was the day of a decidedly naughty purification and fertility festival called Lupercalia. Priests called the Luperci would sacrifice goats and dogs—chosen for their strong sexual drive—and smear the blood on the forehead of two noble youths. Then after having feasts and lots of wine, the Luperci sliced the goat's hide into strips, dipped them in blood, and ran through the streets slapping women with them. The gals eagerly welcomed these blows because they were said to promote fertility and easy childbirth.

Sacrifices and feasts and spanking. Makes our own Valentine's Day pale by comparison, eh?

Let's celebrate our own modern version of this ancient rite. This little history lesson was really just an excuse to introduce the idea of "love taps." We're not talking heavy S&M here: What we mean is a light, quick slap on the fleshiest part of your lover's behind while you're making love. Give your man a light love tap during sex in the Missionary position as you pull him into you. Or ask him to give you a little mini-smack while you're doing it Doggie Style. Hell, you can even ask him to slap his erect penis against your butt a few times. You may both find it very wild and sexy and primal.

If this isn't your cup of tea, skip it, but many people find that these love taps carry a strong erotic charge. Whether it's because the area is already sensitized during sex, or because it touches on buried feelings of power and punishment and permission and taboo, only you can say. Try not to analyze it too much. Instead think about a half-naked hunk lashing you lightly with a soft leather thong—and enjoy!

FEBRUARY

Hear Me

If you want to increase your erotic potential, think about your sense of hearing. As my co-author David Ramsdale says in our book *Red Hot Tantra*: "In our culture, we tend to relegate sound and music to the background—in the elevator, in the car, as the soundtrack for movies or television. When you make love, though, sound takes a place second only to sight. Often there are cues and clues that our brain requires for heightened erotic response." Next time you make love, pay close attention to your auditory environment. Chances are, you're not going to be able to have a very sensual experience if you've got television sitcoms distracting you in the background.

Find out what kind of music most gets you in the mood. Is it rock and roll? Trance music? Classical? How about the exotic, mystic beat of music with an Indian flair? These days, it's not hard to burn a CD of your favorite tunes for seduction and love. Just make sure the music lasts a long time, or put the stereo on repeat. You don't want to be getting up to hit "Play" just as you reach the climax of your own private symphony.

And for goodness sake, if you want to create a romantic mood, make sure your answering machine's turned down and your phone ringer is turned off—or better yet, get voicemail.

FEBRUARY

Snack Break!

Don't forget your taste buds when you're in the bedroom. Keep a glass of your favorite wine or champagne on hand to quench your thirst. However, bear in mind that alcohol is a depressant, and too much can inhibit sexual response in both men and women—so save the guzzling for post-coitus. Have a carafe or glass of ice water nearby, too. Not only will it quench your thirst, but the cubes can come in handy for all sorts of naughty play.

Snacks are nice, too, to help you refuel during breaks in long love-making sessions. Feed each other strawberries dipped in chocolate or slices of tangy fresh kiwi. Drizzle gooey chocolate sauce over your breasts and draw a line down your belly to your pubic area, and ask him to lap it up. Don't forget the napkins or towels. While food can be erotic, rolling around in crumbs isn't. Spread out your repast on a simple tray that can be set aside when you're through eating and ready for more loving.

Don't just gobble your food, either. Try to really taste what you're eating. Let your lover see you savoring every morsel—just like you'll savor him.

FEBRUARY

Position of the Week: Rear Entry, Seated

This is a nice position in which to christen your favorite chair. Just make sure it's sturdy! Have him take a seat while you sit on his lap. The catch is, of course, that you're both buck-naked. Slowly slide down onto his erection, wrapping your legs around the outside of his thighs. (You can also place your legs inside his, although you may find it harder to maneuver.) From here, he won't be able to move much, so you're in charge. Vary your speed as you bounce up and down, rock back and forth, or swivel your hips. If he hasn't had the idea on his own, move his hands to your nipples and clitoris. You can also play with his scrotum and enjoy the lascivious feeling of his rock-hard erection sliding into you.

The *T'ung Hsüan Tzu* calls this position The Goat and the Tree, but it's more fun to call it The Queen and Her Throne!

HISTORICAL NOTE: Today is the birthday of Helen Gurley Brown (1922-), publisher of the groundbreaking, racy women's magazine *Cosmopolitan* and author of *Sex and the Single Girl* (1962).

FEBRUARY

Rear Entry, Solo

There's no reason you can't reap the benefits of the rear entry position without a partner. Get on your hands and knees and use your fingers, dildo, or vibrator to simulate a penis pushing into you from behind. As a variation, lie flat on your stomach and position a thrumming vibrator against your love button as you "take" yourself. If you reach behind yourself, rather than through your legs, you'll be able to angle your fingers downward and have a better chance of stimulating your G-spot. Vary speed and pressure to find out what gets you hottest.

If you've got a suction-cup dildo (see November 13 and 14 for more on dildos), you've got even more options for fun. Attach your dildo to any vertical surface. Slather it with lube, put some pillows under your knees, and slide back onto it. Hold still for a moment to savor the feeling of fullness. As you start to move, enjoy the fact that you're in control of how fast or deeply you thrust! Some lifelike dildos even have testicles, giving you a soft cushion to bounce against. Feel free to pleasure yourself with your fingers or a vibrator!

FEBRUARY

The Sign of the Fish

People born between today and March 20 fall under the sign of Pisces, the fish. Pisceans are caring and sensitive, compassionate and artistic. If you're in a relationship with a Pisces, lucky you: These gentle, dreamy nurturers make wonderful lovers. Seduce him by appealing to his love of fantasy and indulgence. Feed him a wonderfully decadent meal, draw a hot bath, and put your softest sheets on the bed. If you are a Pisces, ask your lover to do the same for you (and throw a nice massage into the mix).

Even if you're not involved with one of these charming sensualists, take a cue today from the Piscean love of fantasy. Today, try writing out one of your favorite fantasies and see what happens. The act of writing has tremendous kinesthetic power. Marry that with the power of your private fantasy life, and you've got the makings of a very erotic experience. Don't worry about literary quality or pass judgment on yourself. Embellish your fantasy as much as you like: The great thing about fantasies is that they give you complete editorial freedom. When you're done, if you haven't already, read your story as you pleasure yourself to ecstasy. Lose yourself in your erotic fantasy dream world. Then put your fantasy in a safe place, or destroy it if you'd prefer. Don't worry: There are more where that came from! Our fantasies provide us with an endless treasure trove of erotic material.

FEBRUARY

Start An Erotic Diary

Today is the birthday of Anaïs Nin (1903-77), the French writer best known for her diaries, published as *The Diary of Anaïs Nin, Vols. I-VI* and *The Early Diary of Anaïs Nin, Vols. I-IV*, in which she talked frankly about her sexual experiences. Her books *Delta of Venus* and *Little Birds* contain some of the best—and hottest—erotica in existence.

In honor of Nin, start your own erotic diary as a way of becoming more familiar with your sexual likes and dislikes. In *Red Hot Tantra*, my co-author David Ramsdale describes how keeping such a diary can help you learn more about what turns you on—and turns you off—so that you can maximize your sexual pleasure. As David rightly states, "How can you ask for what you want if you don't know what it is?" Use your diary to note the surroundings where you make love, your mood, your expectations, techniques used, and orgasmic satisfaction. Have fun with it. Who knows? Reading about your experiences later in the year might turn you on all over again.

Your erotic diary is a good place to track your Sensual Resolutions. Have you tried anything recently that you especially liked, or didn't like? Use your diary as a way to renew your commitment to your sexuality.

HISTORICAL NOTE: Nin's affair with the writer Henry Miller and attraction to his wife June was portrayed in the 1990 movie *Henry & June,* one of the first movies to receive an NC-17 rating.

FEBRUARY

Tantra for Beginners

When most Westerners hear the word "Tantra," they think of esoteric sexual practices that help you make love for hours. In truth, Tantra refers to a body of thousand-year-old Hindu and Buddhist religious practices and rituals. And yes, some of these rituals are sexual. But even these are not so much aimed at helping practitioners (tantrikas) become sexual athletes as to safely awakening the sexual energy inside us. The idea is that when we experience an orgasm, we connect briefly with the Divine. Put simply, we experience enlightenment. So if you've ever described an orgasm as a religious experience, you're not that far off.

This short introduction can't hope to do justice to Tantra. If you're interested, there are numerous books on the market. But today, let's try a very simple Tantric ritual. Get in a comfortable position, lying on your bed, a couch or even the floor. Close your eyes, clear your mind, and become aware of your breathing. Take a deep breath in to the count of six, and then let it out for the count of three. As you breathe in this way, begin to pleasure yourself. Don't force either your breathing or your pleasure, simply note the sensations in your body. Do you feel tingling? Warmth? (Note: if you feel dizzy or lightheaded, *stop.*) After seven to ten minutes, return to normal breathing. And if you want to, go ahead and give yourself an orgasm—if you haven't already!

This is a very simple *pranayama*, or breathing technique, designed to raise your energy and help you focus your mind. Try it with your partner!

FEBRUARY

Sensory Deprivation

Here's an erotic exercise to help you focus on your sense of touch: Take turns blindfolding each other while you're making love. Since you can't respond to visual stimulation, you have to concentrate on your other senses. Get a little Zen about it. If you find your mind drifting, bring it back to what you're feeling in the here and now.

Notice the sensations of your body. How does your lover's mouth feel on yours? How does it feel on your breasts, stomach, and genitals? How does your lover's skin feel against yours? Where does he have hair, and where is he smooth? What do you smell? Trace the contours of his body with your fingertips, and when it's his turn, ask him to do the same to you. As he thrusts inside you, how does your skin feel? What do you experience at the moment you have an orgasm? If you really want to be a little daring, add earplugs. You'll focus on the sensations of lovemaking like never before.

This exercise will also help you think about texture. When you're dressing for seduction, think soft: Cashmere, silk, leather, suede, and velvet. Anything that makes your lover want to touch you gets my vote. Avoid clothes that are confining or scratchy, or anything that's going to make you sweat—unless you don't plan on wearing it for very long.

FEBRUARY

Mardi Gras Madness

The huge celebration that is Mardi Gras is really just one big excuse for partying and carousing before the fasting and self-denial of Lent. The exact date varies from year to year and place to place, but let's celebrate our Mardi Gras today. Since Mardi Gras celebrations are noted for their vibrant and elaborate costumes, have some fun in creating your own erotic masquerade.

Wearing a mask allows you to adopt a different identity, experiment with new roles and personas, and act out fantasies safely. For inspiration, look at the erotic use of masks in movies like *Henry & June* or *Eyes Wide Shut*. Experiment with masks and role-playing in the bedroom. Put on a mask and see what happens. Does it make you feel more uninhibited, freer, wilder? Check out the variety of beautiful and sexy masks on Mardi Gras Web sites like MardiGrasDay.com (www.mardigras-day.com), or head to a costume shop.

But don't stop with the mask. Combine it with a sexy outfit and surprise your lover. Adorn yourself with feathers and beads. Even better, buy some body paints and spend an evening painting each other's bodies. Transform yourself into a spotted leopard or wood nymph, and see whether it brings out your feral nature. Imagine the fun you'll have smearing up each other's designs.

FEBRUARY

Position of the Week: The Carnal Prayer Mat

Here's a graceful twist on the rear entry position. Your partner kneels behind you, his buttocks resting on his heels. Sit in front of him on your heels, so that the soles of your feet touch his knees. Lean forward onto your forearms. The sight you present to him—your delectable derriere and the petals of your labia peeking out from between your buttocks—will be irresistible. As he comes up onto his knees to enter you, lean forward onto your hands and rest your cheek on one or two pillows. This will give you leverage if you want to reach back and caress your clitoris. You can also guide his hand to your sweet spot. Do this in front of a mirror for even more erotic thrills.

To increase the friction on his member, keep your knees and thighs together—and pray that he can last!

FEBRUARY

The Power of Touch

There's nothing like the ritual of a loving massage to help you and your partner relax, reconnect, and get in the mood for love. The simple act of touching each other's bodies, of feeling skin against skin, can heighten anticipation and arousal. As my friend Jane says, "For me, a massage is always key to good sex. A gentle yet aggressive touch using massage oil seduces me and makes me feel warm, comfortable, and deeply satisfied."

You don't need to take classes to give a good massage. Set the stage with soft lighting or candles, relaxing music, and lots of pillows. Have towels on hand not only to dab up excess massage oil, but also to drape over his body if he gets cold. Before touching your partner, warm your hands. Place them gently on his body to center yourself and connect with him. Focus on him, and encourage him to breathe and relax.

Assuming he's lying down, begin with long, flat-handed strokes from his buttocks, up either side of his spine to his shoulders. Circle around and back. Start lightly and increase your pressure. Once he's relaxed, begin working one part of his body at a time. Many people carry their tension in their neck and shoulders, so spend some extra time here. Lean your body weight in as you grasp his muscles and knead out any knots, especially under the shoulder blades. Take your time, and try not to talk other than to check in with him. End the massage with some light strokes over his entire body.

Ask him to return the favor another day—you don't want him to undo all the good you've just done by working on you!

FEBRUARY

Sensual Massage

If the purpose of your massage ritual is arousal, rather than pure relaxation, try these energizing techniques to awaken your lover's senses. When you knead his muscles, use faster strokes rather than slow, deep ones. Open-handed chopping movements down the back will break up tight knots and wake up his muscles. Use these percussive moves on fleshier parts of his body; on bony areas, tap with your fingertips instead. Run your fingernails in light circular movements across his scalp. This feels great!

Then, switch to firm, feathering strokes. Starting at his scalp, run your fingers down his body, around his earlobes, neck, insides of his arms, chest, belly button, inner thighs, calves, and toes. Tease his penis with a "barely there" touch. Lighten the stroke each time until you're barely touching him, and you'll sense the energy coursing between you. If you have some real ostrich or peacock feathers, this is the time to bring out them out. Graze his skin ever so lightly, and he'll be shaking with anticipation by the time you're done.

FEBRUARY

Relaxation Is for Genitals, Too!

Isn't genital massage just masturbation? No. The point of genital massage is therapeutic—to release tension that's built up there—so that you can enjoy lovemaking more fully. Ever heard of muscle memory? Just as your body remembers how to perform physical skills like walking, bicycling, or skiing, it also remembers trauma like falls, blows, and other stresses. Your genitals retain not only pleasurable memories of attraction and ecstasy, but negative experiences like rejection as well.

You can massage your genitals yourself. Warm your hands, and before you begin, put one hand on your heart and the other covering your vulva. Then, working from your belly button, gently massage in circular motions down to the pubic mound and upper thighs. Working on each side at the same time, knead your outer labia and then your inner lips with a gentle pinching motion. Put your thumbs on either side of your clitoris and work your way in tiny circles down your entire vulva. Be careful around your urethral opening, especially if you have massage oil on your hands. Slide a fingertip into your vagina, pressing around the edges of the opening, and gradually work your way in. Take your time. When you're done, lie quietly for a moment so that you can give yourself a chance to deal with any emotions that may arise. And if you're aroused, go for it!

LEAP YEAR BONUS If this is leap year, extend your genital massage to self-pleasuring or lovemaking with your partner. Note how the genital massage has affected your sexual response. Do you feel more relaxed? Is it easier for you to achieve an orgasm?

CHAPTER THREE

MARCH

"March comes in like a lion and goes out like a lamb."
—Proverb

We've all heard that old saying about March. Now let's see how sexy we can make it. This month's tips will show you how to bring out your inner lioness— the sexy, ferocious part of you that's aching to be let loose. We'll also tap into the joys of gentle, joyful lovemaking in honor of spring's new beginning.

In the Victorian language of flowers, giving someone March's birth flower, *jonquil,* symbolized a request to "return my affection." Place jonquils around your home as a reminder to show love not only to your partner but to yourself. And that includes showing yourself affection through self-pleasuring!

For a bonus, wear this month's birthstone, *aquamarine,* which is said to bring love and devotion. Legend has it that it can even reawaken love in a long-term marriage!

MARCH

Get to Know Your Inner Kali

The Hindu goddess Kali, consort of the god Shiva, is the Queen of the Night in Hindu mythology. She represents our dark side, our hidden fantasies, the push-pull of our fascination with what's kinky and taboo. She personifies raw, unbridled, aggressive sexual passion. She's a royal bitch—and she lives inside each one of us, screaming to get out. She *wants* you to experience the power of sensual ecstasy in *all* its forms.

Tonight, take some time to get in touch with your inner Kali. As you pleasure yourself, imagine that you are sexually all-powerful. What would you do? What kind of sexual experiences would you have if there were no shame attached and you were totally in charge? Would you be an empress with legions of hunky servants at your sexual beck and call? A dominatrix with men quivering at your feet? Would you have men fighting over you, with your body as the prize? As you approach your orgasm, be detailed. Be explicit. Your mind is the perfect place to explore a sexual power trip. It doesn't mean you're going to do it. Besides, the chances are good that there are thousands of other gals out there with fantasies more extreme than yours. Kali tells us that even our darkest fantasies are part of us. Get to know them, and claim their power—and yours.

MARCH

A Walk on the Dark Side

Let's take another day to find out what Kali has to teach us. For one, she wants us to shine a blazing torch into the dark room that holds our forbidden fantasies. She wants us to indulge in these thoughts without shame.

Yesterday, we imagined being all-powerful. But maybe you fantasize about being submissive, restrained, or even raped. So many women have these fantasies that there's no need to feel embarrassed. If that's your fantasy, indulge it—especially today. As you masturbate, or even when you make love, let your mind wander to your wildest, most over-the-top outlandish fantasies. Do you fantasize about taking on an entire squad of Canadian Mounties? Or perhaps having your lover perform oral sex on you in a movie theater while strangers hold you down? Your mind is the safest place to explore these thoughts, no matter how outrageous you think they are.

Having a colorful erotic fantasy life is healthy and fun, and real women do it. As my good friend Connie says, "No fantasy is too outrageous, illegal or unreasonable when I'm masturbating or making love. If the visual of a trapeze, the motorcycle driver who smiled at you in the parking lot, and a bottle of ketchup are leading you down the path to nirvana, don't analyze it or tear it apart—keep it going. The mind is a wonderful film projector of what really turns us on. Don't shut down the production studio mid-action!"

Tonight, don't put any limits on your erotic fantasies. Don't judge yourself. As Kali shows us, sexual pleasure is natural. And shame is overrated.

MARCH

Position of the Week: Woman on Top

This position isn't called the "Cowgirl" for nothing. Men love to watch a woman "ride" them. You get the benefits of being in control of the speed, rhythm, and angle of your thrusts—and of deep penetration, if that's what you want. He gets to rest on his back and feast his eyes on your beautiful breasts, the uninhibited passion on your face, and his erection disappearing into your warm wetness.

Don't just hop on him, though. Take charge and warm him up with some woman-on-top foreplay. Straddle him gracefully, and stay on your hands and knees as you tease him by brushing your hair or the tips of your erect nipples over his body. Bestow passionate kisses on every inch of his skin, then grasp his erect member in one hand and use it to caress your belly and pubic mound. Rub it against your clitoris. Wet it against your moist inner lips and the entrance to your vagina. Tease him by slipping him inside you a tiny bit and then pulling out. When neither of you can stand it anymore, slide ever-so-slowly onto his anxious member. As you move faster and faster on top of him, give him some squeezes with your toned PC muscles. Ride 'em, cowgirl!

HISTORICAL NOTE: Today is the birthday of Jean Harlow (1911-1937), American film actress and sex symbol known as the "Blonde Bombshell."

MARCH

Speak Up, I Can't Hear You!

Your voice is the most reliable tool you have to ensure sexual satisfaction. If you like what's happening, speak up! And if you don't like what's happening, that's all the more reason to make your desires known. Believe it or not, most people don't have ESP, and though moving his hand (or other body part) gently to where you want it can be a nice way to give advice, there's nothing wrong with just *telling* him you want him to move a little to the left when he rubs your clit or whatever. Chances are that he'd be relieved to get a little guidance. "Communicate, communicate, communicate," a male friend advises. "My girlfriend has trouble having an orgasm through intercourse. She needs direct, heavy clitoral stimulation. She also likes anal stimulation and penetration as well. I wouldn't have known this unless I asked. I'm constantly asking if this feels good or what she needs, and vice versa."

You don't have to be a drill sergeant, and don't criticize. Some gentle verbal direction in your throatiest purr, followed by a moan of delight, might be all the instruction your willing pupil needs.

So let's practice. Next time you're making love, *tell* your man at least one thing you'd like him to do to rock your boat. If it's something you've always been shy about asking for, you get a gold star! When he hits the spot, let him know. A breathless "Yes! Right there!" or "That's it!" are words every lover craves.

MARCH

The View from the Top

Since we're focusing on the woman on top this month, let's talk about what to do once you're there. The good news is that you control the action. You can put your hands on either side of his shoulders, or hold onto the headboard to give yourself even more leverage. You can even pin his hands to the bed to give him a taste of pleasurable powerlessness. Or you can simply sit straight up. (Those of you who've had horseback riding lessons can imagine "posting.") Squeeze your thighs around his pelvis as you bounce up and down. Let him see you playing with your nipples—or take his hands in yours and guide them to your breasts, or his thumb to your clitoris. Reach back and caress his balls and inner thighs. You'll send shivers up his spine.

Meanwhile, take advantage of the view. Look down at his staff sliding in and out of you, a view it's hard to catch in missionary. Feast your eyes on his excited face. Notice how his chest gets flushed as he approaches an orgasm—this is your cue to slow down if you want to draw things out. You're in charge of the pace. You can encourage him to thrust up against you, or demand that he lie still as you ride him to heaven!

MARCH

An Orgasm a Day? How About an Ecstatic Moment a Day?

The goddess Kali represents woman's sexuality in its wildest, most liberated incarnation, as well as her capacity for infinite pleasure. This pleasure is yours for the taking. You don't have to wait for the "right" moment: You can access this pleasure any time, any place, either alone or with a partner. Take a page from Connie, a thirty-five-year-old self-described "lover of life" who makes seizing ecstasy part of her daily experience.

"Every day, I have at least one ecstatic moment, even if it's not an orgasm," she says. "And if I don't have a lover at my fingertips, then I play with myself. These times may come during any time of the day. I've had many a climactic, ecstatic moment with myself in public restrooms, hidden cubicles, remote tables in the library—anywhere I could really get it on with my mind and my fingers. Of course, the possibility of being caught is a turn-on just as much as getting away with it. I have a very active imagination, so I can drum up any style of fantasy at a moment's notice and come quickly with great satisfaction and bliss."

Like Kali, Connie claims unbounded pleasure as her birthright. In Indian art, Kali is often portrayed nude, symbolizing her freedom from false consciousness and illusion. She loves spontaneity and authenticity. So if you feel lustful, like Kali and like Connie, go with the flow. Honor your libido. The ecstasy you feel may just bring you one step closer to enlightenment! At the very least, it will put a big smile on your face.

HISTORICAL NOTE: Today is the birthday of Elizabeth Barrett Browning (1806-61), the English poet and early feminist whose *Sonnets from the Portuguese*, written in secret to her husband before they were married, is one of the most beautiful collections of love poetry ever written.

MARCH

Take Charge of Your Pleasure

Don't be shy about touching yourself while you're on top. Unless he's some kind of control freak, he'll love the idea that you're so consumed with passion that you can't keep your hands off your love button. And besides, men love to watch women pleasuring themselves. Try different positions to see which one gives you the best access to your pleasure zone. Is it sitting straight up, with his hands on your hips to steady you? Leaning forward and bracing yourself on the bed, so that you can slide your fingers between your bodies? If you usually use a vibrator to achieve an orgasm, use it now. He may enjoy the buzzing sensations as well.

He may also be able to rub you with his thumb from this position. Take his hands and put them where you want them. You can even keep a hand on top of his to show him the right speed and pressure. As you're getting close to coming, move faster and faster on him. Again, when you're on top, you control the pace!

MARCH

Your Move

Believe it or not, men do *not* always like to be the ones to initiate sex. Sure, at the beginning of a relationship, some men enjoy the pursuit, and some women enjoy being pursued. That delicious uncertainty, on both sides, is what makes our hearts race during the mating dance, but after a while, *always* being the sexual initiator can get a little old. This may come as a shock to some women, but *men are human, too.* Can you imagine how exhausting it would be, night after night, if *you* had to be the one to suggest sex? If *you* were always the one to risk rejection? Everyone likes to be desired once in a while.

I'm not saying you have to tackle your guy in the living room, although that could certainly be fun. Be yourself, but make your desires known. While you're at a party, whisper in his ear that you want to make love to him. Wake him up by exploring his nether regions with your mouth. Climb onto his lap—naked (don't do this during the last two minutes of the championship game, unless you want to understand what sexual rejection feels like). And when all else fails, try the direct approach and grab his package. He'll get the hint.

MARCH

Tie Him Down

On March 5, we discussed pinning his hands to the bed while you're on top. If you and your partner have absolute trust in each other, you can take this a little further. Get out some silk scarves, a tie, or stockings to *lightly* tie his hands above his head or to the bedpost. The point isn't to truss him up like a turkey—the "bonds" should be light enough so that they don't cut off the blood supply and he can easily slip out of them. The thrill is mostly psychological: You're reducing him, temporarily, to a helpless prisoner of your passion who is "forced" to enjoy your lust without raising a finger (literally). Take advantage of it. Rub your body all over his. Stroke and suck him until he's begging you to take him. After you've both had your pleasure, untie him right away, because otherwise his muscles will get stiff and uncomfortable.

There's absolutely nothing weird about experimenting with a little "light" bondage, which we discuss in greater detail on October 26. (Actually, there's nothing wrong with experimenting with the heavier versions, if that's what gets you off *and* you know what you're doing.) You're simply exploring the many different aspects of sexual power in a safe, fun way.

MARCH

Position of the Week: The Race of the Member

The *Kama Sutra* calls this posture The Race of the Member, probably because you'll be racing to keep his member from beating you to an orgasm. In this position, he draws his knees up to his chest, while you lower yourself onto him, sitting on the backs of his thighs. Once again, you're in charge, because he won't be able to move much, although he can help you by putting his hands around your waist or under your buttocks to facilitate your strokes up and down on his shaft. He can also wrap his legs around your waist.

Unless you're gymnasts or exceptionally limber, you may not be able to stay in this position for very long. And he may feel pinned to the bed like a lab specimen—which, in a way, is the point. With him helpless on his back, you get to dominate him for a little bit. Let your powerful sexual urges surface, and chances are, you'll be on your way to a more powerful orgasm.

HISTORICAL NOTE: Today is the birthday of Sharon Stone, a versatile actress whose roles have ranged from bombshells to Wild West gunslingers to the caring mother of a physically disabled boy. Her performance as the dangerous, sexually uninhibited Catherine Tramell in the 1992 movie *Basic Instinct* in many ways embodied the spirit of Kali.

MARCH

Self-Loving Reason #3: Come Again, and Again, and Again

Let's state the obvious. If you know how to make yourself come, the chances are that you'll come faster and more often, with or without a partner. Do the math. The majority of women—anywhere from fifty to seventy-five percent—*do not* achieve orgasms through intercourse alone because they don't get enough stimulation of their love button during penetration. The hands-free orgasm is generally a myth perpetuated by lazy men; chances are, everyone's going to have to pitch in. By engaging in regular self-loving, you'll be better able to tell or show your lover what to do—or take matters into your own hands, so to speak. (Most guys love to watch a woman touch herself. Trust me.)

Besides, by playing in your own garden, you're free to experiment and expand your orgasmic repertoire, further increasing your opportunities to experience the Big O. While many of us have a tried-and-true way to bring ourselves off, variety ensures that you won't be dependent on one technique as your body and situation change over the years. You'll multiply the ways in which you can experience pleasure. And that's nothing to sneeze at.

MARCH

The Pleasure Principle

Why do we feel sexual pleasure in the first place? Your brain and body work together during foreplay and arousal like a well-rehearsed orchestra to prepare you for showtime. As you touch each other, receptors on your skin get all hot and bothered. These receptors send signals to the reflex center in the lower part of your spinal cord, which in turn tells the muscles around your genitals to relax and go for it. And go for it they do. Blood flows into your genitals and pelvic area. Your vaginal lips swell and redden; your vagina becomes lubricated, more elastic and elongated; and your clitoris and nipples harden. You may get a "sex flush" across your upper chest and neck. His penis stands at attention. As your arousal heightens, your clitoris retracts under the clitoral hood. It hasn't disappeared, and you should keep up whatever you're doing.

While your conscious mind is thinking, "Where did I stow the condoms?" your autonomic nervous system goes into overdrive. Your skin gets pinker and more sensitive; your heart beats faster; and your breathing speeds up. Meanwhile, your hypothalamus releases a quartet of hormones and chemicals into your bloodstream. Adrenaline makes you alert and sensitive, oxytocin helps you feel emotionally attached to your partner, endorphins give you a feeling of well-being, and dopamine triggers a giddy mélange of love and attraction. Is it any wonder that love is compared to a drug? It truly is a natural high!

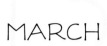

MARCH

Anatomy of an Orgasm

What exactly happens when you experience the Big O? First of all, the mechanisms that cause you and your man to experience an orgasm are pretty similar, except that his climax is usually accompanied by ejaculation. (Yours might be, too: See March 15 for a discussion of female ejaculation.)

Here are the details, for the next time you're caught short of cocktail party chat. During arousal, the relay of nerve signals in your body escalates to the point when release is inevitable. Your breathing becomes shallower and quicker, and your body stiffens. Then it's time for the fireworks: Your body suddenly releases all that accumulated sexual tension by having an orgasm. For men, muscle contractions force semen into the urethral bulb at the base of the penis. (This is the point of no return.) The muscles of the urethral bulb and the penis start to contract as well, forcing the ejaculate out. In women, levels of oxytocin soar to a peak, stimulating the muscles of the vagina to contract rhythmically. The uterus also contracts in waves, from the top down to the cervix.

In both men and women, the muscular contractions of an orgasm occur at 0.8-second intervals and usually last for several seconds. When the contractions stop, the orgasm is over, but the good feelings aren't. Enjoy the afterglow, that post-orgasmic feeling of profound relaxation sweeping over your body. Yummy.

MARCH

Press On!

Let's take a mid-month break from being on top with what the *Kama Sutra* calls The Pressed Position. Draw your knees back toward your chest, only instead of staying curled up like a bundle, or resting your legs on your shoulders, press the soles of your feet against his chest, a gesture that can be as intimate as putting your hand on his heart. Encourage him to massage and fondle your feet for an erotic mini-reflexology session. Meanwhile, caress and stroke his thighs. Your man might want to rise up on his knees while he's inside you to give him better leverage.

Since your clitoris will be hiding between your thighs, you might experience a little less stimulation, so you might want to fondle yourself or ask your lover to give you a hand, so to speak. He'll also need to be gentle with the depth and vigor of his thrusts, as your vagina will become shorter at this angle. You may feel quite vulnerable in this position, which can be a turn-on. Don't worry: You'll have a chance to turn the tables later.

MARCH

Nectar of the Goddesses

A fair number of women emit an odorless fluid right before or during an orgasm, especially with G-spot stimulation. If you're one of these women, relax! There's nothing to worry about. Research has shown that it isn't pee, but a substance that's often referred to as female ejaculate. There's still debate about what's going on—because this response varies so much between women, it's hard to study—but basically, here's the deal. The spongy tissue around your urethra contains glands similar to those in the male prostate (which is why the ejaculate is sometimes called female prostatic fluid). Like the prostate, these glands produce an odorless fluid, and this fluid is what's ejected through the urethra during the contractions of an orgasm. The amount varies. Some women spurt; others leave a wet spot; and others may not notice anything at all.

In ancient times, female ejaculate was considered sacred. Aristotle wrote about it, as did the second-century Greek physician Galen. It's also featured in ancient Japanese and Chinese erotic art, as well as the *Kama Sutra.* So think of it as your own hot love nectar, have a few towels on hand, and just enjoy.

MARCH

Go with the Flow

If yesterday's discussion of female ejaculation has left you inspired, there are a few things you can do to feel more comfortable about—and even encourage—your flow of lust liquid. (Keep reading, but you have to promise not to burden yourself with another sexual expectation. Some women ejaculate, some don't. If you fall into the latter group, don't sweat it.) To take the pressure off yourself, practice alone before you try this with a partner, and take your time.

First, keep doing your Kegels. A strong PC muscle translates into stronger ejaculation. Next, do whatever it is you do to arouse yourself. You may even want to come a few times so that your pelvic muscles are fully relaxed. Then, begin stimulating your G-spot until you're really hot and bothered. When you feel yourself climaxing, bear down—that is, push down and out with your vaginal muscles—as if you were giving birth. And then *let go*. If you've gone to the bathroom, you won't pee. (And if a few drops of urine escape, what's the big deal?) You may actually want to practice stimulating your G-spot when you have to urinate, and then letting it flow, so you get used to the feeling. When you're ready to try the real thing, empty your bladder, get out a few towels, and make sure your love geyser has lots of room.

MARCH

Position of the Week: Orgasmic Role Reversal

The *Ananga Ranga* describes woman-on-top positions as *purushayita-bandha*, or role-reversal positions. The guide states that they are to be used when the man needs a rest or hasn't yet satisfied his partner. Clearly the author considered a woman's sexual needs just as important as a man's! In the Orgasmic Role-Reversal Position (*purushayita-bhramara-handha*), for example, you'll definitely take charge. With your feet on either side of his hips, squat onto his thighs and ease his penis into you. Close your thighs firmly and move in a churning motion. The stated goal is for the woman to "thoroughly" satisfy herself. So do what you need to do!

While this position takes a little bit of balance—not to mention strong thighs—it allows you to control the angle, speed, and depth of penetration as you circle over him. It's not bad for toning the quads, either, although if you get tired, he can help you out by putting a hand under each of your thighs. This will also keep you from losing your balance (see March 18 on why this could have disastrous consequences). Just grip tightly with your thighs, and you should be fine.

Kalyana Malla, the author of the *Ananga Ranga*, compares the woman in this position as a "large bee." Whatever! Just imagine you're hovering over his throbbing stem, and pollinate away.

MARCH

Prevent Penile Mishaps

Yes, being on top gives you a chance to ride him like a lust-inflamed cowgirl. But that doesn't mean you can throw caution to the wind. While it's very unlikely you could hurt a man during sex, if you do move too quickly on top of him, you could bend and tear the two tissue chambers inside the penis. To avoid this rare yet painful phallic accident, make sure you're fully lubricated when you hop on. And if he slips out, don't just bounce on him hoping he'll slide in. Ouch. Pause, and use your hand to glide him back inside you.

If by some freak mishap his little man does get injured, you'll know right away. Mr. Stiffy will become not only become Mr. Softy, but it will also turn black and blue and swell up. Get him to the emergency room *immediately*. Failure to do so could cause problems down the road, which could put a big crimp in your love life.

MARCH

More Ways to Play with the G-Spot

Last month, we introduced the G-spot. This month, explore other ways to experience its delights. There are a variety of vibrators and dildos designed especially for G-spot exploration and stimulation (see December 13 for more on these toys). You'll find them curved at the end to reach where fingers often can't. Many online sites even have a special category for G-spot vibrators.

Get your partner in on the G, too. Most men have heard about the G-spot, and they're typically just as confused as women. That's why knowing about your own sweet spot can help you explain it to your lover. (Men have a urethral sponge around their urethra, too—it's what gives them a hard-on.) Many women find that rear entry intercourse hits their G-spot just right. Being on top might also help you control the angle at which his love shaft strokes your inner walls. Ask him to use one of your new G-spot toys on you, or his finger and eager tongue.

MARCH

First Day of Spring

Finally, winter is over, and it's the first day of spring! In parts of the Middle East, March 20 is actually considered New Year's Day; Iranians, for example, celebrate Norooz, or "new day," on this date. With this in mind, create your own special rite to welcome the new season. Steal away for a night at a bed-and-breakfast in the country, or your favorite romantic inn.

If you can't get away for a whole night, fill your home with spring flowers and plan a living-room picnic. Take a long luxurious bath together, then lie down on the bed and exchange a few small, sexy tokens of affection for each other. Think of naughty gifts that will encourage you to get busy, like a romantic game or a pleasure kit filled with massage oil, body powder, and whatever other flirty little novelties strike you. Ring in the new season by spending the entire evening in bed—talking, cuddling, and making love.

MARCH

Ramming Speed: Aries

People born between March 21 and April 19 fall under the sign of Aries, signified by the ram. Ruled by the planet Mars (named after the Roman god of war), Arians are said by astrologers to be competitive, courageous, and often stubborn. They can also be impulsive, with an affinity for adventure and risk. Arouse your Arian lover by engaging him in an exciting game of tennis or even a lusty debate. To an Aries, this is foreplay! Don't be afraid to suggest new positions or techniques: An Aries will love being kept on his toes. If your sign is Aries, you'll enjoy athletic, physical sex, especially this month's woman-on-top positions.

Here's one to try from *The Perfumed Garden*. When he's on his back, have him spread his legs and put a pillow under his hips. Slide onto him, keeping your thighs pressed firmly together and your legs out behind you. Push up with your arms—kind of like an X-rated pushup—and move up and down. By gripping his penis tightly with your vagina and thighs, you increase the stimulation on his member. You can also maneuver so that your clitoris is stimulated, too. Be like the ram, and be stubborn about getting the pleasure you deserve.

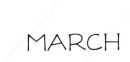

MARCH

The Half-Pressed Position

For a variation on March 14's Pressed Position that will produce some very interesting sensations for both of you, stretch one leg out past his side while you keep your other foot pressed to his chest. This "half-pressed" position gives your clitoris a better chance of making contact with his body; if not, either of you will be able to fondle your love button. He also has room to run his finger in light strokes along your inner thighs and vulva.

If your leg gets tired, you can wrap it around him, resting your calf and foot against his back and buttocks. This has the added benefit of giving you more leverage. Vary the depth of your thrusts and swivel your hips as you arch against him. Because this position constricts the vagina, he may need to thrust more gently. Just remember that we're in the "goes out like a lamb" part of March, so immerse yourself in the tenderness of the moment.

MARCH

Bath Toys

On February 2, we talked about the pleasure a well-placed stream of water can provide you in your very own bathroom. But if the pressure of the water isn't enough to send you on the wet path to an orgasm, check out the variety of waterproof vibrators on the market. The amazing selection ranges from standard, smooth cylindrical vibrators to G-spot toys to jelly vinyl shafts. Check out Web sites like MyPleasure (www.mypleasure.com), Good Vibrations (www.goodvibes.com) or the Xandria collection (www.xandria.com). The Aqua Touch Vibe, for example, fits on your finger and comes with three different sleeves for variety! Imagine the fun you'll have soaking in a relaxing bubble bath after a hard day as you massage your erogenous zones. Don't forget the lube. Silicone-based lubricants stay slick in the water.

You can enjoy bath toys with a partner, too. Try a slimmer waterproof toy, like the Tsunami, a smooth, ice blue G-spot vibe that sparkles with silver glitter. Run the vibrator over his inner thighs and shaft, or, if your bathtub is small, see if he'll sit outside the tub and pleasure you. After you've enjoyed your own tidal wave of pleasure, you'll surely be able to think of some way to float his boat.

MARCH

Position of the Week: Reverse Cowgirl

Next time you're on top, ride him a little differently. Instead of facing him as you slide down onto his erection, face away from him, so that you're looking at his feet. Not only does this give both of you some new sensations, but it also gives him a nice view of your beautiful buttocks. In fact, *The Perfumed Garden* suggests leaning forward and putting your hands on his thighs or the bed in a position termed Reciprocal Sight of the Posteriors. (Just be sure not to lean too far forward, or you could cause him some pain.) Not only does this give him an even better view of your derriere, but he might also get a glimpse of his member plunging in and out of you, a sight guaranteed to turn on any man.

While you're here, take advantage of the scenery: caress his inner thighs and testicles, and even yourself! You can also "milk" him with your PC muscles in a trick that the Kama Sutra calls The Mare's Position. Whatever you decide to call it, when you're in the Reverse Cowgirl, you're sure to lasso yourself a rollicking good time.

MARCH

Full-Body Kissing with a Tease

Here's a variation of the full-body kissing game you played on January 20. Explore each other's bodies with kisses, but leave out the rating scale. Instead, take turns slowly kissing each other everywhere *except* the genitals. When it's your turn, you can stare at his member, breathe on it, lick around it—everything except touch it. By the time you're kissing the soles of his feet, his shaft will be standing at full attention, and he'll be begging you to release him from this exquisite torture. Then it's his turn to do the same to you. Repeat at will.

It's up to you how you determine the "winner." For example, the first person who breaks down and kisses the other person's sex could be the "loser." Of course, as in all erotic play, "losing" is a relative term, and you can have fun deciding the "prize" between the two of you before you start.

MARCH

Pleasure Begins at Home

We've already talked several times about the joys of self-pleasuring, and hopefully by now you've realized that self-loving is one of the keys to year-round sexual ecstasy (and if you haven't, we'll keep giving you one reason every month). Maybe you're fully comfortable touching yourself, but maybe you've been too shy or unsure of how to proceed. Everyone can use a refresher. Besides, the more techniques you know, the more variety you can bring to your self-love life.

Obviously, there's no "right" way to masturbate: It's really whatever makes you feel good. Some women like deep, strong pressure; others want no direct touch at all. Here's a way to get you started (or ease you into your preferred method). Cup your hand as if you were about to do the royal motorcade wave. But instead of greeting the adoring throng, say hello to your pubic mound by placing your hand lightly over it. Then move your entire hand in circles, touching your clitoris gently with the heel of your hand, then the sides, then your fingers. Try different pressures, and moving your hand at varying speeds. You might also try this over your panties. Fantasize that your hand belongs to an eager lover who's panting to get to third base. You decide whether to go all the way, but my vote would be yes.

MARCH

Slip Slidin' Away

One key ingredient for sex with yourself is lubrication. Using a little of the slippery stuff is nicer on your delicate tissues and makes it easier to warm up if you're trying to rev your own engines from a complete stop. By mimicking your body's natural arousal, you'll make it easier to achieve the real thing.

One of the nicest things about lubrication is that there are so many options available, including your own natural juices, saliva, K-Y jelly, and water- or silicone-based lubricants. Although some sex books will tell you otherwise, avoid oils, whether vegetable- or mineral-based. If they get into your vagina, they can stay there for a while, inviting bacteria. Also, scented massage oils contain alcohol, which can irritate your tissues. And Vaseline, which is hard to wash out of your body, is best avoided altogether. If you're embarrassed about buying lube in a store, go online. Any of the Web sites mentioned on March 23 will carry a wide selection.

To get the most out of your lubricant, start with just a little bit. You can always add more later. Pour a small amount on your fingertips, and as you begin to pleasure yourself, luxuriate in the slippery, sensuous feeling of your fingers on your moist, delicate tissues. One nice technique is to rub your clitoris for a while, then dip a finger into your vagina to sop up the wetness growing there, and use your own juices as a naturally sexy lube on your aroused bud.

MARCH

Hey Diddle Diddle

As you turn yourself on, vary your routine by trying different techniques, pressures, and speeds. Gently massage your love button in various directions: Side-to-side, up and down, and in circles. Speed up and slow down, or keep up a continuous pressure. Try lightly tapping yourself or giving your love button delicate love pats. Pulsate your fingers as fast as you can, imagining that your hand is an exotic vibrator. Try stroking down from the top of your pubis over your outer labia, barely touching your clitoris. Tease yourself. Have some fun.

Which brings me to my next point. Relax. Yes, orgasms release tension and indeed, people often masturbate for the release alone, but if you're new to self-loving or having trouble achieving orgasms, it helps to start from a relaxed state of mind. Turn off the phone and television. Leave distractions—thoughts about work, financial worries, relationship problems—outside the bedroom door. Slow down your breathing—it will speed up anyway as you get aroused—and imagine your breath traveling to the tips of your toes and back up. A warm bath is also a good way to ease tight muscles as you ease your hand between your legs.

MARCH

Tie Me Up, Tie Me Down

At the beginning of the month, we talked about bringing out your inner Kali. There are other ways to explore your darker side: Explore the flip side of being in power. The March 9 tip described how a little light bondage for him can increase the thrill for both of you. Again, assuming you have complete trust and faith in each other—in other words, do *not* do this with one-night stands—let him tie you up lightly. By the way, being submissive is *not* the same as being passive: You can still let him know with your moans and cries and the gyrations of your hips that you like what he's doing. Beg him to release you from this exquisite agony by plunging his staff inside you.

Any time you're engaging in bondage of any sort—no matter how much you trust your partner—make sure you have a "safe word." This is a word or phrase that means, unconditionally, *Stop now*. It shouldn't be a word like "stop" or "untie me," which, in some sex games, can be seen as part of the fun. Make it something like "red." Your partner *must* immediately stop what he's doing and/or untie you, or you have every right never to see him again!

MARCH

"If absolute power corrupts absolutely, does absolute powerlessness make you pure?"
—*Harry Shearer (1943-), American actor and writer*

Giving It Up

Just because you like to give up control and be tied up once in a while doesn't mean that you're terribly kinky or, heaven forbid, politically incorrect in your sexual desires. You're just exploring a different aspect of sexuality. By being submissive, you temporarily give yourself completely to another person. Kind of romantic, if you think about it. It can also be freeing—you're relieved of responsibility or guilt for anything you're made to do. It might even give you "permission" to experience a more intense orgasmic release if there's nothing you can do about it. Plus, even though you're a slave to someone's whim, you're also the sole focus of his attention, which can be pretty darn exciting.

Here's a fun variation on yesterday's tip. Have him tie your hands and feet together lightly while you're on your hands and knees. He then takes you from behind as you struggle vigorously against your bonds—pushing back wildly against him, of course, and enjoying every second of it. After he releases you, he can massage your wrists and feet, and more, just as I'm sure you did for him when it was his turn to experience the bonds of love.

MARCH

Position of the Week: Inverted Embrace

As March goes out like a lamb, let's look at a more tender way for the woman to be on top. In the Inverted Embrace position of the *Ananga Ranga*, you lie outstretched on top of him, pressing your breasts to his, and grasp his waist as you move in all directions: Up and down, side-to-side, and in circular motions. Because you're skin to skin and heart to heart, this position can be quite intimate, even though you're in control of the movements. In fact, you may enjoy the feeling of power that this brings. The *Ananga Ranga* says that women-on-top positions are "especially useful when he, being exhausted, is no longer capable of muscular exertion." Your man can lie still and rest, of course, but chances are he'll have plenty of energy to respond to your movements.

Focus on your breath and see if you can synchronize your breathing with his. Feel his heart beating against yours. Unlike other woman-on-top positions, this one lets you bestow gentle butterfly kisses on his face and deeper, soulful smooches on his lips. What a nice way to end the month!

CHAPTER FOUR

APRIL

"Sweet April showers / Do spring May flowers."
—Thomas Tusser (1524 -1580), English farmer and writer,
A Hundredth Good Points of Husbandrie

The Romans called this month Aprilis, from *aperire* ("to open"), no doubt because this is the month when the new buds of flowers begin to bloom. This month's tips will guide you through your own sexual blossoming, with suggestions for awakening your senses after the cold of winter. Or take a page from the early Anglo-Saxons, who named April *Eostre* or *Eastre* (Easter) month, after the Teutonic goddess of spring and fertility, whose festival they celebrated on the day of the vernal equinox. The Easter bunny, a symbol of fertility, is a holdover from this tradition. Some experts believe the Eostre is actually a variation of Inanna, the Sumerian goddess of procreation, love, and war. You may not be ready to procreate literally, but let your imagination fertilize your sexual creativity.

Fill vases with April's birth flowers—*daisies*, signifying beauty and innocence, and *sweet pea*, symbolizing delicate pleasures. Let the blossoms remind you of the beautiful pleasures in store, and approach your lovemaking with new eyes.

April's birthstone, the *diamond*, has long been a symbol of love and is said to have powers of protection, courage, and strength. If you can't afford a real diamond, hang a crystal in a window to reflect the clear spring light.

APRIL

April Fools!

Mark Twain said, "The first of April is the day we remember what we are the other 364 days of the year." Having a sense of humor is a critical success factor for any relationship, whether it's with a partner or with yourself! Today, find a way to make each other laugh, whether it's by playing an affectionate practical joke on your lover or sharing the funniest thing that ever happened to you in bed. "Looking foolish does the spirit good," author John Updike commented.

Besides, the old adage that "laughter is the best medicine" actually appears to be true. A study conducted by the University of Maryland Medical Center suggested that laughter, along with an active sense of humor, may prevent heart disease. More recent research has found that unlike fake orgasms, fake *laughter* actually makes you feel better: The body doesn't know the difference between phony and real laughter, and releases endorphins anyway—the same hormones your body releases during sex. Laugh during sex, and you get a double dose.

Many researchers believe that laughing helps us bond to each other. So watch a comedy together: Films like *Tom Jones* are both sexy and funny. Check out a book like *Sex and Humor: Selections from the Kinsey Institute.* Play a game. Act silly. Laughing is sexy, and that's no joke.

APRIL

Shake Yourself Out of the Doldrums

With spring in full swing, how can you be in a sexual rut? Simple. Even couples who are crazy about each other can too easily fall into the same old bedroom routine. First you kiss, then his hand goes there, your hand goes there, you perform some mouth music on each other for three minutes apiece, and then you make love in the missionary. While I'm not knocking either the missionary or doing whatever you know turns you on, a little variety is the spice of life.

So today, surprise him. Change your sequence. If your man doesn't know what's coming next, he'll stay excited and focused. Instead of making love at your usual eleven p.m. (when you're both apt to be most tired), grab him when you get home from work. Wake him up for a sleepy morning quickie. Have pre-date sex instead of post-date sex. Interrupt the action mid-coitus for some oral loving. Instead of letting him mount you as usual, flip over and beg to be taken from behind. Be creative and do whatever you can to get out of your old lovemaking-by-the-numbers pattern.

HISTORICAL NOTE: Speaking of shaking things up, today is the birthday of author Camille Paglia, whose provocative writings on culture and sexuality challenge both liberals and conservatives. Her 1991 book *Sexual Personae: Art & Decadence from Nefertite to Emily Dickinson* explored the connections between art and pagan ritual. Giovanni Jacopo Casanova (1725-98), the Italian writer and adventurer whose name has become synonymous with that of the legendary Don Juan, was also born today.

APRIL

Bounteous Breasts

As a symbol of both fertility and sexuality, the female breast has received more than its share of attention throughout history. But have *you* given your girls the devotion they deserve? Today, stand in front of the mirror and get to know your knockers. Your breasts probably aren't the same size or shape, they may not point in the same direction, and your nipples may sprout a few hairs (most women's do). Like you, your orbs have their own monthly cycle: They may be smooth right after your period; sexually sensitive in the middle of your monthly cycle, when estrogen levels are highest; and swollen and tender right before your period. Throughout the month, pamper them with sunscreen and lotion. And explore their sensual possibilities to the hilt.

Most women's breasts and nipples are extremely sensitive to touch; a few lucky women can even climax from nipple stimulation alone. Today, start by massaging your breasts and nipples by inscribing languorous circles on them with the palm of your hand. Start out lightly, barely touching your skin, and gradually increase the pressure as your nipple hardens. Try different speeds and directions. Squeeze them gently, or knead them more roughly. Take note of the delicious electricity radiating through your body. And know that your breast size has nothing to do with your ability to feel lots and lots of pleasure.

HISTORICAL NOTE: Celebrate the birthday of Marlon Brando (1924-2004) today by checking out his performance as Paul in the 1972 film *Last Tango in Paris*, one of the first sexually explicit mainstream films.

APRIL

Be Nice to Your Nipples

Your nipple protrudes from a circular, pigmented area known as the *areola*. Both areolas and nipples come in a variety of shapes, sizes, and colors. Today, focus on your nips to find out what kind of pressure and treatment makes them stand at attention. Massage them. Pinch them. Roll them between your thumb and index finger. Pull them. Jiggle them. Wet your fingers and stroke them across your rosy nubs. Graze them lightly with your fingernails. Lean over and play with them; this sends blood to the region, increasing the sensitivity of both your breasts and your nipples.

As you play with your nipples, hold out for as long as you can without touching your pubic area. Then see what happens if you tease your nipples as you pleasure yourself: Most likely, you'll double your ecstasy.

Let your partner watch you engage in nipple play. Chances are, he'll be begging to help out, but if not, feel free to give him a hint. Tease him by letting him touch your breasts only through your shirt, as though you were a couple of teenagers. Once your shirt's off, encourage him to lick, suck, and kiss your breasts and nipples. Keep going until neither of you can take any more.

APRIL

Nipples: His Turn

Time to wake up your man's nipples as well. Some men love to have their nipples stimulated, and some can't stand it. The only way to find out is to dive right in. First, warm up his chest area by massaging his pecs from the outside in, toward his nipples. This will send the sensation directly to his little nubbins until they're standing at attention. Now, lick gently with your tongue, flicking his nipple into hardness, and then blow softly on it. The feeling of cool air on moist skin will make him shudder with delight. Just don't go on for too long, or pleasure will turn into pain.

If he seems to be up for it, you can follow your tongue action with your front teeth—gently—but be very, very careful: you're nibbling, not munching. You might even want to cover your teeth with your lips. After a little of this—again, don't carry on too long—switch to your hands. Pull lightly on each nipple, then both together, with light tugs of your thumb and forefinger. If he likes it, add a little twist. Make sure you use enough pressure that he can feel it, but not so much that you send him into agony. Gauge his reactions as you increase the pressure.

APRIL

Glorious Glutes

Filled with sensitive nerve endings, the buttocks are an oft-neglected erogenous zone. Give them the attention they deserve, and you won't regret it. Run your hand over your own behind, stroking, massaging, or squeezing it as you see fit, especially when you're pleasuring yourself. Alternate between light strokes and gentle kneading. Caress it with lace or silk. And next time you're with your man, show him what you want him to do by guiding his hands to massage your enticing derriere. Men not only love to look at but touch your booty.

Many men also like to have their own bottoms burnished by a good massage. Put your thumbs in the middle of each of his globes with your other fingers fanned out towards his hips. Stroke and knead his glutes with firm motions, moving your thumbs in circles with increasingly less pressure until you're barely touching him. Then squeeze each buttock in turn. When you're done, he'll be not only relaxed but turned on.

Don't forget his butt during sex, either. Men find it extremely sexy when you grab their glutes to pull them into you. Because the bottom is so sensitive, he might also get off on a few quick, light "love taps" in the middle of one of his cheeks. If he likes it, go for it. If you're lucky, he'll do the same for you!

APRIL

Position of the Week: Butterflies in Flight

Taoism is an ancient Chinese system of religious and philosophical thought dating from the fourth century B.C. The Taoists believed that sexual intercourse was a natural, healthy part of life that brought into balance the opposite and complementary forces of yin (female) and yang (male). They collected their sexual wisdom in explicit guides called "pillow books," the most famous of which is *T'ung Hsüan Tzu* by Li T'ung Hsüan, who describes twenty-six positions for lovemaking in evocative and sensual language.

The beautifully named Butterflies in Flight is a simple variation of the woman-on-top (also known as The Unicorn's Horn) position. Insert your lover's Jade Stem into your Coral Gate and lie on his body, breast to chest, your thighs and feet resting on top of his. Grasp his hands in yours and stretch out your arms from your sides like butterfly wings. As you move up and down, push with your feet. Your movement will be limited, as is his, but you'll enjoy nice skin-to-skin contact—including friction against your Jewel Terrace (the Taoists' name for the clitoral area) as you undulate on top of him.

APRIL

Skin Games

The skin is the largest organ of your body. With thousands of sensory receptors per square inch—even more in your fingertips and lips—your skin is designed to respond to the lightest caress. With the advent of spring, it's time to reawaken the sensitive nerve endings that have been hidden under layers of winter clothes.

Assemble a variety of fabrics—everything from soft materials such as silk, fur, and velvet to rougher textures like wool or terry cloth. Blindfold your partner, undress him and stretch him out on the bed, gently spreading his legs. Tell him that he must let you do anything you want to him. Make sure the bedroom is warm: The only goosebumps you want to cause are by your touch.

Now graze his skin with each fabric, teasing them gently across his face, chest, belly, and inner thighs, down to his legs and toes—everywhere *except* his genitals. All he has to do is lie quietly and focus on the sensations (threaten to stop everything if he moves—the anticipation will drive him wild). Finally, caress his erogenous zones with the materials you've used on the rest of his skin. You decide when and how you want to release him from this sensual torture. Then it's your turn! (See April 15.)

APRIL

Your Love Button

There's much more to your clitoris than the little love button you see at the spot where your labia meet. First, take a look. The clitoris varies from woman to woman and day to day in size, color, shape, and the amount it protrudes. And no, it doesn't "disappear" when you get aroused; it just might seem that way when surrounded by engorged labia or when it retracts slightly during an orgasm (in other words, when somebody's doing something right). When you pull back the hood of skin covering it, you'll see the clitoral glans, the sexual organ that corresponds to the head of the penis. Approximately 6,000 to 8,000 nerve endings are concentrated here, more than in any other structure in the human body.

If you press down above the clitoral glans, you'll feel the clitoral shaft, a rubbery cord that leads up to the pubic bone. The clitoral shaft separates into two legs called *crura*, which extend like a wishbone for about three inches on either side of the vagina. Two more extensions, the clitoral bulbs, branch off from the shaft underneath each inner lip. These consist of erectile tissue that fills with blood when you're aroused—just like the erectile tissue of the penis, only there's more of it in the clitoris.

Why the anatomy lesson? Well, the more you know, the more fun you can have. Because the clitoral network extends throughout the genital area, you stimulate it indirectly even when you're stimulating the urethra, vagina, or anus. So make friends with your clitoris. It's the only organ in the human body whose sole purpose is to transmit sexual sensation. What's not to love about it?

APRIL

Beware Orgasm Typecasting

Thanks to Hollywood, the porn industry, and trashy romance novels, a lot of men and women think a woman "should" be able to climax through vaginal intercourse alone. Bollocks. The vast majority of women require direct clitoral stimulation to achieve orgasms. Find out how your clit likes to be stimulated, and you increase your chances of climaxing exponentially.

That's not to say that women don't have different types of orgasms: You may feel something quite different if you climax during G-spot stimulation than you do when you come through masturbation of your clitoris alone. Some researchers suggest that this is because different nerves connect different parts of your genitals to your brain. And of course, some women may climax during breast play, Kegels, or even just by thinking racy fantasies. Heck, it's even possible to have an orgasm in your sleep. The point is that there's no "right" way to achieve an orgasm.

Take a moment to look at whether you've been guilty of orgasm typecasting. Do you think of a certain type of orgasm as better than another? Do you get frustrated if you can't describe every orgasm as "earth-shattering"? See if, just for today, you can stop ranking your orgasms. To paraphrase Gertrude Stein's line that "rose is a rose is a rose," an orgasm is an orgasm is an orgasm. It's a subjective experience. Know what gives you pleasure, and own it.

APRIL

Self-Loving Reason #4: Guilt Begone!

Many of us were brought up to feel guilty about masturbation, even though it's something that almost everybody does. If you don't believe me, ask the Kinsey Institute, which found that ninety-four percent of men and at least seventy percent of women masturbate! In fact, we have sex researcher Alfred Kinsey to thank for removing the stigma around masturbation. He debunked the Freudian notion that it was an "immature" activity, noting that in fact, it was masturbation that most likely allowed women to achieve orgasms. Since then, sexologists like Betty Dodson, Lonnie Barbach, and Shere Hite have promoted the joys of self-loving. In 1972, the American Medical Association even proclaimed masturbation a "normal" sexual activity.

Still, it's hard to get rid of some of those deeply ingrained taboos. Even worse, it's hard for many of us to enjoy pleasure guilt-free, especially sexual pleasure. (When was the last time you ate a piece of rich chocolate cake and *really* enjoyed it, despite its undeniably delicious taste?) So let's dive right in, because the more time you spend with your body, the more you'll see that the experts are right: Self-pleasuring is natural and healthy. Just for today, give yourself permission to masturbate and to experience an orgasm in your favorite way. You'll feel good and be more relaxed, which means you'll probably be nicer to the people around you. And why feel guilty about that?

APRIL

Encourage Bed Head

Since we're focusing on awakening our senses, let's start at the top. As Vatsyanyana noted in the *Kama Sutra,* hair can exert a powerful influence over lovers. There's nothing like the feeling of your man running his fingers through your hair, stroking it, fondling it, moving a wisp tenderly out of your eyes. Return the favor, and then some. Give him an erotic scalp massage or shampoo, moving your fingertips—and fingernails, if that feels good to him, which it probably will—in circles over the crown of his head, over his temples, and down. Gently pulling at his hair might feel great as well. A good, vigorous scalp massage can have him eating out of the palm of your hand. Why do you think people love getting their hair washed at the salon or barbershop?

Use your clean, beautiful locks to your advantage, too. If your hair is long enough, make your man lie still and focus on the sensations as you brush your hair along his naked body. Hold your body above his so that only your hair makes contact with his skin as you tickle him with it everywhere. Wind it gently around his penis, let it unravel, and then brush it across his shaft and scrotum.

A final note: After lovemaking, don't jump up to brush your hair. There's really nothing sexier than hair that's been mussed by a passionate roll in the hay.

APRIL

Praise for Your Pubes

Whether you shave, wax, or go bare, your pubic hair (or lack of it) is another part of your body that can be put to good use. Make him lie on either his back or stomach as you trail your public hair over his body, brushing it against his skin. Rotate your hips in luxurious circles, or move them back and forth. The feeling of your soft bush and the growing wetness inside it will drive him wild. It can also be nice to fondle each other's pubic hair before, during, and after lovemaking. Stroke it tenderly; you can try pulling on it, but be gentle.

A few words about pubic hair grooming. A *Glamour* magazine survey of nearly 3,000 men found that their preferences were almost evenly divided when it came to hair down there: Thirty-eight percent preferred a trimmed, tidy but natural-looking bikini line, thirty-two percent thought a woman looks best completely bare except for a "landing strip," twenty-five percent liked the area totally bare, and five percent like their women natural. The upshot? Do what *you* like, but if you find he has a preference, give it a try.

To wax or shave? Waxed hair tends to grow back softer and finer, but it can get expensive. However, note that if you shave, be sure you're freshly shaved before getting intimate. You don't want to give his member—or his face—razor burn.

APRIL

Position of the Week: Side-by-Side Clasping

Side-by-side positions encourage you to relax and take it slow, allowing you to touch and stroke your lover instead of racing toward the finish line. They also come in handy if you don't have much room to maneuver; if, for example, you're stuck in a single bed or a one-person tent. With the Side-by-Side Clasping Position, the *Kama Sutra* suggests that the man lie on his left side and the woman on her right as you intertwine your outstretched legs around your partner's.

Of course, you can lie on whatever side feels comfortable. Take your time to caress each other's face and body. This position is nice for new partners: Wrapping yourself around your lover is a highly comforting way to quell the anxieties of a burgeoning sexual relationship. And established partners will enjoy the chance to express tenderness in this unhurried, gentle manner.

Doing it side-by-side offers several advantages. Penetration is shallow, so although he may not be able to thrust deeply, he should be able to last longer, and your cervix will get a break. Friction will also be a factor. In fact, if he slides up the bed, there's a chance his penis may even be able to rub against your clitoris. You can vary this position by wrapping your top leg over his hip and around his waist. The *Ananga Ranga* calls this The Crab Embrace.

APRIL

More Breast Fun

Since this month is all about awakening your senses, let's take another day to explore your breasts' sensitivity to pleasure. Ask your lover to blindfold you and rub your breasts and nipples with different materials—satin, silk, velvet, and fur—as you guess what they are. Of course, you get a "prize" for every right answer. As you get better at guessing, he can graduate you to more textured materials, such as lace, wool, or even a soft Egyptian cotton towel. Have him caress you and tweak your nipples wearing leather gloves or rub them with a soft natural hairbrush.

Ready for round two? Move on to organic substances. See how it feels to have him daub your nipples with whipped cream, honey, or melted chocolate. Blindfolded, your senses will be exquisitely focused, and of course, you'll both enjoy his licking them off. Play with the feeling of cold against your warm skin. Have him circle your nipples with an ice cube until they stand at attention. Daub them with a warming massage oil or cool peppermint oil. It goes without saying that everything he does to you, you get to do to him.

A final note: You can—and should—try today's sensory experiments by yourself to develop your own erotic sensory awareness.

APRIL

Awesome Areolas

Whether it's you or your lover playing with your breasts, don't neglect your areola, the sensitive, pigmented tissue that surrounds your nipple. Whether they're small or large, coffee brown or rose pink, your areolas are richly endowed with nerve endings—maybe even more so than your nipples. So make the most of them. Give them the same attention you give your nipples. Encircle them with a moistened finger. Encourage your lover to paint delicate spirals on them with his tongue. See if stimulation of your rosy rings alone makes your nipples stand at attention and sends shudders of pleasure down to your clit.

The tiny bumps around your areola are hair follicles, and they can be quite sensitive, too. Run your finger over them, enjoying the sensations. By the way, it's entirely normal for you to have tiny hairs here. Just pluck them away and don't worry about it.

If you're feeling saucy, daub some rouge onto your areola and nipples and see how sexy they look peeking out from behind sheer lace or a bra with the nipples cut out—or simply bare, waiting for your lover's touch.

APRIL

The Root of the Problem

According to Tantra and similar systems of thought, there are seven major energy centers, or *chakras*, stacked in a column from the base of the spine to the crown of the head. When they are aligned, they allow the life force (also known as *chi* or *prana*) to flow freely. The first chakra is the root chakra, located in the perineum, the point between your anus and your genitals. As the literal root of the body's energy system, it's related to survival and overall vitality. A closed root chakra translates into fear, insecurity, and sex without pleasure. (Ever heard of someone called a "tightass"? They've got a closed root chakra.) Opening your root center can reconnect you to the earth, balance and ground you, and reduce your insecurity and fear so that you can enjoy lovemaking more.

While there are many ways to open the root chakra, today we're going to look at one that can help you enjoy more sexual pleasure. Ground yourself by standing up straight and relaxed, your feet shoulder width apart and your knees bent slightly. Meditate on your root chakra, and imagine a small red flame of energy there, burning away your fears and filling you with energy. Stimulate this chakra by contracting your PC muscle as you breathe in deeply, and releasing as you exhale with a quiet "ahhhhh." Visualize this squeezing as "sealing" the energy into your body. Rock your hips back and forth as the heat moves up through your body. To finish, imagine the flame subsiding to a warm glow at your root. Imagine it there while you make love.

APRIL

In Praise of the Prostate

Assuming your man enjoyed the back door play on January 30, here's a way to take it a bit further and send him over the edge: Prostate massage for men. First, a few words about the prostate gland, that little internal organ that produces ejaculatory fluid. It's located close to the root of the penis and is comparable to your G-spot, and like the G-spot, it can produce incredible pleasure when stimulated. Some men can come from prostate massage alone.

As with the January 30 tip, make sure you have lots of lube on hand, and spend some time warming up his member with either your mouth or your hand (he's more likely to enjoy it if he's turned on). When he's good and ready, slip a finger into his anus about two or three inches and crook it forward toward his pubic bone. You'll feel a little bulge about the size of a nut. Stroke it with a come-hither motion, and you'll stimulate the bulb of his penis and his prostate at the same time. If you do this while you're sucking or stroking his penis, you'll give him an orgasm that he'll forever describe as "mind-blowing."

HISTORICAL NOTE: Today is the birthday of Humphrey Verdon Roe (1878-1949), the English aviation pioneer who founded, with his wife Dr. Marie Stopes, the first birth control clinic in Britain.

APRIL

Start Foreplay Early

One way to awaken your senses for passionate lovemaking is to start foreplay early—*really* early—before you're even in the same room together. Don't forget that anticipation can be one of the biggest turn-ons! Just think about the early days of your relationship, when you could hardly wait to see each other, and your imagination ran wild with what you'd do when you were together. There's no reason you can't re-ignite that spark with a little mental foreplay.

Call him randomly during the day and tell him exactly what you're going to do to him later. Describe in detail the loving ministrations you'll bestow with your tongue upon every inch of his body, including his erect penis; or how you're touching yourself, thinking of him; or how you've just had this incredible fantasy that you have to share with him. Put his brain into sexual overdrive. When you get off the phone, he won't be able to wait to "get off" with you in person.

You can also put technology to good use. Most cell phones today let you send short text messages. Because they have to be short, text messages are a great way to get right to the X-rated point.

APRIL

Position of the Week: The Spoon

Turn that early-morning cuddling session into something more racy. In this position, you're lying side-by-side, your back to him, curled together like two spoons in a drawer as he enters you from behind. Penetration may not be very deep in this position, but this means he might be able to last longer. You can change the angle by stretching your top leg back over his or bending forward at the waist. Guide his hands around to stroke your breasts, stomach, and clitoris as you grind your pelvis against him. The pressure of your thighs around his member will create some nice sensations for him as well.

To allow your man to thrust more deeply, bend your knees and encourage him to tuck his knees in behind you as he clasps your hips for leverage. You might also take a page from Tantric techniques by seeing if you can synchronize your breathing. Imagine the energy from his heart flowing in through your back to your heart, and back again.

Snuggling with your lover in the spoon position can be very comforting. What a nice way to wake up!

APRIL

Bullish on Taurus

If you or your lover were born between today and May 20, you fall under the sign of Taurus, an earth sign symbolized by the bull. Ruled by the planet Venus, Taureans are stable, patient, and affectionate people who are deeply attached to their homes, friends, and families. They are also very sensual.

Taurus is an earth sign, so earthy is the name of the game. Whether you or your partner is a Taurus, find ways to make your lovemaking last. This month's side-by-side positions give you lots of time for kissing and caressing. Think natural, think nudity, think sensual, and you'll be thinking like a Taurus.

Or cook a sensual (but not too heavy) meal. It has been said that the way to a Taurean's sex organs is through his stomach. Rent the movie *Tom Jones* and study the chicken-eating scene, then cook a meal that allows you to demonstrate orally what you'd like to do to your man. You may just end up on the table as dessert.

If neither you nor your partner is a Taurus, use today as an excuse to practice your oral skills. You'll find lots of tips in this book to help you brush up. Toro, toro, toro!

APRIL

More Mental Foreplay

Don't save all your X-rated talk for the phone. Next time you're out in public—at a party, in line at the movies, in a café—whisper salacious nothings in his ear. Tell him explicitly what you have planned for him later that evening. This is even more exciting if you keep a straight face, so that others have no idea what you're talking about. For all they know, you could be discussing the weather. Instead, you're driving him crazy with randy talk that for the moment, he can't do anything about.

Can't think of what to say? You can always resort to that tried-and-true technique of confiding in him that you "forgot" to wear any underwear. It should be true, naturally, at which point you can guide his hand to your derriere so he can see and feel for himself. He'll spend the entire evening picturing what's under your skirt. Of course, make sure your skirt isn't so short that *everyone* can see you're not wearing panties. It may have worked for Sharon Stone in *Basic Instinct*, but in the real world, it's a little tacky. Put your imagination—and his—to work.

The idea is to use anticipation as an aphrodisiac. Chances are that it will get you both hot and bothered, and dying to get your hands on each other in private. Engage the brain, and pretty soon you'll have all five senses on high alert.

APRIL

Awakening Your Sense of Sight

By appealing to your lover's five senses—sight, smell, taste, hearing, and touch—as well as your own, you awaken your bodies and prepare them for extraordinary lovemaking. Finding creative ways to engage your senses will help you stay in the moment and blossom into a more sensual person.

First, let's take our sense of sight. Human beings are visual creatures, particularly men. In Tantra, sight relates to the chakra in your solar plexus, and to the element of fire, so give yourself and your lover visions that will arouse your passions. One of the surest ways to do this is to look at erotic pictures together, especially nudes or portrayals of people having sex. You can find these easily in men's magazines, or, if your tastes are more highbrow, in books of photography such as *Erotique: Masterpieces of Erotic Photography* by Rod Ashford; *Eros,* by Linda Ferrer and Jane Lahr, which mixes beautiful prints with classic erotic poetry; and *Love Lust Desire: Masterpieces of Erotic Photography for Couples* by Michelle Olley. Delve into the past with *Eros in Pompeii: The Erotic Art Collection of the Museum of Naples* or *Eastern Erotica: Chinese, Indian and Japanese Eroticism in Art and Literature.*

After thumbing through some of these books together, you'll be anxious to duplicate the images you see. Or simply use the photographs and drawings as inspiration for your solo erotic fantasies.

HISTORICAL NOTE: Today is the birthday of Vladimir Nabokov (1899-1977), author of *Lolita*, which portrays the involvement of a middle-aged man with a sexually precocious young girl, whom he terms a "nymphet."

APRIL

Awaken Your Sense of Smell

In Tantra, the sense of smell is associated with the root chakra, which governs survival and the instincts. Smell is also one of our most primal senses. That's why titillating your olfactory nerves through the ancient art of aromatherapy is such a potent way to arouse your erotic energy. Anoint your body, bath, or bedroom with essential oils such as rose, jasmine, or lavender. In particular, aromatherapists often recommend ylang-ylang and sandalwood for their aphrodisiac properties. Be careful, however: Essential oils are highly concentrated, so don't put them on the skin undiluted, or you may cause a skin irritation. Dilute them with a "carrier" oil such as almond, olive, or sunflower.

Here are two games you can play to heighten your sense of smell. Light one or two candles in your bedroom or another comfortable room. Keep the room dark so you focus on scents and not sight. Blindfold your partner, and pass essential oils under his nose. (Don't stick the bottle directly under his nose; a mere whiff should be enough.) Let him inhale and enjoy the scent before going on to the next one. He'll be tantalized wondering what's coming next.

Next, while he's still blindfolded, tell him to smell you. Lay back while he inhales the clean body scent emanating from your neck, breasts, and thighs. He can pretend he's a wild animal, sniffing for his mate. Then switch roles.

See February 13 for more ideas on how to use smell to your sensual benefit. Or check out Web sites like Aworldofaromatherapy.com or aromaweb.com.

APRIL

Awaken Your Sense of Taste

Tantrics believe that taste connects to your second, or sexual, chakra. Take special care with the foods you consume before getting romantic. Light foods are best if you're planning (or hoping for) a night of passion. Think about it: After a big heavy meal, most of us want to sleep, not sex it up. So plan your menu accordingly. In addition to having yummy snacks on hand to re-stoke your fires during a long bout of lovemaking, use the following technique to heighten your sense of taste. Again, blindfold your man or ask him to close his eyes as you place bites of sweet foods like mangoes, kiwi, or chocolate truffle on his tongue. Whet his thirst with sips of wine or champagne. Let him savor each taste before you move on to the next one. Then switch places.

There are several foods that can act as aphrodisiacs (at the very least, they're fun to play with). Feed each other seedless grapes, plums, or figs. (An open fig is thought to represent the female genitals.) At dinner, let him see you suck on an asparagus spear or take a banana into your mouth. (Remind him that bananas contain lots of potassium and B vitamins, needed for sex hormone production.) Chocolate contains phenylethylamine, the chemical your body produces when you're in love, as well as antioxidants. Combine a chocolate truffle with a glass of Merlot to double your pleasure. Oysters have been documented as an aphrodisiac since the second century A.D. They also contain lots of protein, and zinc, which increases potency. Have fun planning your menu!

APRIL

Awaken Your Sense of Hearing

In Tantra, hearing is associated with the throat chakra. It is also related to the sacred sense of awareness, which is awakened by sound. Like our sense of sight, hearing stimulates our hearts and our imagination, especially our sexual imagination. Think of the effect that your lover's voice has on you when you hear him on the phone. Stop sometime and listen to his breathing, the beating of his heart, or the rain on the roof.

Put your ears to good use. Read each other some erotic bedtime stories from the annual *Best American Erotica* and *Herotica* series, or anthologies like *Erotic Edge: Erotica for Couples* and *Sweet Life: Erotic Fantasies for Couples.* Heck, you can even try *Penthouse Letters* or *The Story of O.* The racier, the better.

You can also buy many erotica anthologies on audiocassettes or CDs. Or check out CDs like *Cyborgasm* or *Cyborgasm 2*, which contain not only erotic stories, but recordings of real sexual encounters as well. And speaking of recordings, try taping your next encounter—with his permission, of course. Listening to it later may just get your fires burning once again.

Back on February 16, we talked about selecting music to enhance the mood. Another thing to try is a sound machine. These feature digital recordings of natural environments, from babbling brooks to ocean surf, that help you create a serene environment or transport you to your own exotic getaway, where you can imagine waves crashing on a white sand beach, all in time to your lovemaking.

APRIL

Awaken Your Sense of Touch

Tantrists believe that touch is connected with the heart chakra, which nourishes love and compassion. That's why our lover's lightest touch can send shivers down our spine. Massage is great, but there are types of touch that will awaken your senses and his. Turn the entire body into one big erogenous zone:

+ Ears: Don't just jam your tongue into his ear canal and blow like a hurricane. Nuzzle his lobe and gently lick all around it, then blow lightly.

+ Eyelids: Bestow gentle butterfly kisses on his lids. Flutter your own eyelashes over his skin.

+ Neck: Kiss, suck, and lick the area under his ear and jaw. Run your tongue lightly over his Adam's apple.

+ Belly button: Kiss him in circles around his stomach, working your way in a spiral to his belly button, then point your tongue and stick it in and out.

+ Back: Kiss your way insistently down his spine to his tailbone, where lots of sensitive nerve endings gather. Run your tongue along the crease of his buttocks.

+ Inner thighs: Starting at the knee, kiss upwards toward the place where his upper thigh meets his pelvis. Avoid his penis until he's begging. Some people find the back of the knees erotic, too.

+ Feet: Suck on his toes. Lap your tongue gently over the soles of his feet. Don't forget his heel, which is considered an erogenous zone by some.

By the time your mouth finishes its tour of his body, he'll be warmed up and ready for action, and hopefully he'll have picked up a few ideas to try on you!

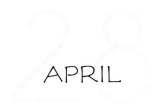

APRIL

Position of the Week: The Scissors

This position takes some finesse, but it's a lot of fun. Lie on your back while your man lies behind you on his side and enters you. Now maneuver yourself around so that your body is at a ninety-degree angle to his, and swing your top leg over his hip and your bottom leg between his thighs. In this position, he can penetrate you more deeply, and also fondle your clitoris. (If he can't reach, you can do it for him.) And while his genitals receive new, interesting stimulation, your hands are free to fondle each other. It's an interesting way to do it from behind comfortably and still have the opportunity to make eye contact.

A variation on this position is to lift both your legs as he enters you from behind and at a right angle. You may have to bend your knees, but again, this gives you lots of room to stroke each other.

APRIL

Over the Rainbow

So the scissors wasn't acrobatic enough for you? Try a position that *The Perfumed Garden* calls The Rainbow Arch—or alternately, Drawing the Bow, for reasons you'll soon see. Start out lying side-by-side with him behind you. Now, scoot slowly around so that your top leg goes over his hip while your bottom leg goes under him, while he keeps his legs together and enters you (essentially, you'll be looking at his feet). Reach out and hold them for leverage as he thrusts (or tries to thrust) against you. Meanwhile, he can hold your shoulders or your waist.

Sure, you may not be able to stay like this for very long, but it's fun to try creative positions like this every once in a while. And it might produce some interesting sensations—as he plunges his arrow into you, you may indeed feel like you're about to take flight!

APRIL

Intro to Vibrators

Hopefully, this very sensuous month has left you with a fertile imagination, heightened your senses, and showered you with ideas to get your libido blossoming. In preparation for May, let's get playful with some very adult toys.

From handheld massagers to jelly-filled vibrating dildos, today's vibrators offer a variety of ways to slake your sexual thirst. Many women have experienced their first orgasms with these pleasure toys, which provide the unflagging stimulation that they need to achieve climax. Unfortunately, the many positive reasons for using vibrators have been obscured by a haze of misinformation, misconceptions, and negativity. Let's try to clear up some of the confusion. First, there's no need to worry that your vibrator will "replace" your man or that you'll become addicted to sex toys. On the contrary, by helping you learn how to pleasure yourself—with or without a partner—and explore the full scope of your sexuality, vibrators open the door to enjoying other types of sexual activity to the utmost.

Besides, the more orgasms you have, the easier it will be for you to reach your climax. Who cares how those orgasms come about (no pun intended)? Besides, let's face it—vibrators feel great, and thanks to the Internet, they're easier to buy than ever before.

There are a million different ways to enjoy vibrators, and we'll be talking about some of them in the coming weeks and months. You're only limited by your imagination in how you put this information to use. In honor of April, remember to keep an open mind.

CHAPTER FIVE

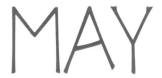

"*The month of May was come, when every lusty heart beginneth to blossom, and to bring forth fruit; for like as herbs and trees bring forth fruit and flourish in May, in likewise every lusty heart that is in any manner a lover, springeth and flourisheth in lusty deeds.*"
—*Thomas Malory, English writer,* Le Morte d'Arthur

Named after Maia, the Roman goddess of spring, May marks the reappearance of spring flowers in all their glory—and encourages lovers to indulge in all sorts of naughty deeds. That's why this month's tips suggest getting out of the house for a little love *al fresco* on May Day, or driving him wild with some creative handwork.

But the fun doesn't stop there. Good Vibrations, the famous San Francisco sex store, has designated May National Masturbation Month. So this May's tips will feature a special focus on self-loving!

Fill your home with May flowers like *hawthorn*, symbolizing hope, and *lily of the valley*, which the Victorians used to represent a return to happiness, which certainly seems appropriate as spring bursts forth. Find a way to incorporate *emerald*, this month's birthstone, into your surroundings as well. Signifying love and success, emeralds are said have soothing and healing properties.

MAY

May Day!

Today, create your own May Day celebration by dancing around his maypole—outdoors. There's something inherently delicious about making love *al fresco*. Perhaps it's the feeling of having fresh air kiss your naked body, or the freedom of communing with the elements and the object of your lust at the same time. Maybe it's just the thrill of possible discovery.

Pack a picnic and your lover into a car, and don't let him know what you have planned. Wear a flowing skirt and no panties. If you leave *some* clothing on, your activity will be less obvious if someone stumbles upon you in the act. Seek out an isolated (but safe) spot like a remote state park or a beach that doesn't get many visitors. Set up your "picnic" blanket where you'll be able to see or hear if someone's approaching. (Don't forget to bring an extra blanket in case you need to cover up quickly.)

Feed your lover seductively from your picnic basket to get him in the mood. As you start feeling frisky, remove a piece of your clothing, and dare him to do the same. Do whatever you need to entice him to go all the way. Lose yourself in the unique locale, but use your judgment as to whether you want to go the Adam and Eve route and undress entirely.

NOTE: Be careful when you pick the place for your open-air tryst. A conviction for indecent exposure or lewd conduct will put a real damper on your love life.

MAY

Self-Loving Reason #5: It's Healthy!

In honor of Good Vibration's National Masturbation Month, let's talk about yet another great reason for rubbin' your nubbin: It's good for your health. Don't believe me? Then listen to the experts. In 1972, the American Medical Association finally came right out and stated that masturbation is a "normal sexual activity." No doubt, they were thinking of the many health benefits of self-pleasuring:

+ It tones and strengthens your vaginal and pelvic muscles
+ It increases the blood flow into the pelvis, helping your body fight yeast infections
+ It flushes the prostate gland, reducing your man's risk of developing prostate infections
+ It releases endorphins and chemicals like oxytocin into your bloodstream, giving you a feeling of well-being
+ It fights menstrual cramps and PMS
+ It relieves stress (more about this later)
+ It gives you a great cardio workout
+ It's the ultimate in safe sex!

And those are just the *physical* benefits. We haven't even gotten into the mental and emotional benefits. For example, a recent study discovered that elderly men who masturbated experienced less depression than those who didn't. So today, just remember that all those myths about masturbation as being bad for your health are just that—myths. And keep your fingers crossed (when they're not busy paddling the pink canoe) that one day we'll pick up the paper and read about a study promoting self-loving right next to the article advocating a daily glass of wine. At least after masturbating, it's safe to drive!

MAY

If You've Never Had an Orgasm or Want to Have More

You've never made the acquaintance of the Big O? Don't feel bad. You're not alone. Therapists will tell you that you're "pre-orgasmic": It's not that you *can't* have an orgasm, you just haven't had one *yet*. Here are some tips to help you get started, or, if you're a seasoned self-pleasurer, to help you give yourself a masturbation makeover:

+ **Do your homework.** Check out do-it-yourself books like Lonnie Barbach's *For Yourself* or *Sex for One* by Betty Dodson, or videos like Dodson's *Selfloving*. Or visit Web sites like Clitical.com (www.clitical.com).

+ **Make time.** Some programs recommend that you devote an hour a day for several weeks to self-pleasuring. If that seems daunting, block out some time every few days. You certainly can have some fun naming the appointment in your Palm Pilot.

+ **Get yourself in the mood.** Find some way to be completely alone. Turn off your cell and turn off the ringer on the phone. Check any residual guilt at the door. Let your mind wander. Read erotica or watch videos to fill your mind with sexy images.

+ **Foreplay: It's not just for partners.** Get yourself warmed up. Stroke your breasts and thighs. Squeeze your nipples. Massage your vulva. Don't expect to go from zero to sixty in five seconds.

Take your time until you feel randy. Then *stop* for today. Yes, you're a tease. Tomorrow we'll delve into some specific techniques for bringing yourself to the edge and plunging over. Bet you can hardly wait to be alone with yourself again.

MAY

If You've Never Had an Orgasm or Want to Have More: Part II

So you've put the moves on yourself using yesterday's warm-up techniques, and now your mind and body are all hot and bothered. What next? Time to go to third base, and maybe even all the way. Try the following:

+ **Get to know yourself—even better.** Begin stroking your genitals and experimenting with different moves: One finger or two; your palm; your knuckles. Repeat whatever feels especially good. Rock your pelvis.

+ **Breathe.** You'll feel stronger orgasms with deeper breathing. Of course, if holding your breath works better for you at first, go for it. But experiment with your inhalation and exhalation.

+ **Start and stop.** It's okay to start and stop, especially if you have trouble letting go. Take a little break, and then start again. Steady stimulation can sometimes actually desensitize you. Stopping and starting may get you closer to achieving an orgasm.

+ **Don't try too hard.** If you start to get frustrated because you get close and then lose it, stop for a while, then build up again slowly. Forget about having an orgasm as a goal. Just enjoy the ride.

+ **Don't let up!** As you get closer to achieving an orgasm, your clitoris will get harder. Press or massage more firmly. Once you start to climax, keep stimulating yourself until you're too sensitive to keep going. You may have a more intense orgasm, or maybe even a second one.

How will you know if you've had an orgasm? Oh, you'll know. Your genitals will get all swollen and wet, you'll feel steady contractions in your vagina, and your entire body may tingle. You may not experience fireworks the first time, or every time, but don't be disappointed. There's always tomorrow, and the next day, and the next....

MAY

Position of the Week: The Yab Yum Position

Yab Yum, which means "the union of father and mother," is the classic Tantric sexual position. It does lend itself to spiritual experiences, and it's ever so easy. Your man sits on the bed or the floor—or the ground, if you're enjoying an erotic *al fresco* picnic—as you lower yourself onto him and wrap your legs around his waist. He can cross his legs below you in the lotus position, or stretch them out. Place your right hands at the base of your partner's spine as he does the same. Look deeply into each other's eyes. Kiss, but keep your mouths and tongues still for a moment while you concentrate on sharing each other's breath. You may not be able to move much, so focus on the slow tilting movements of your pelvis, accompanied by deep squeezes of your love muscle.

Tantrists believe that vertical positions such as these allow the energy to rise up through your chakras, or energy centers, allowing you to experience expanded consciousness and more intense, blissful orgasms. Your mileage may vary, of course, but whether you practice Tantra or not, there's no doubting that the Yab Yum position is extremely intimate and loving. Like all sitting positions, it allows you to make lots of meaningful eye contact as you kiss and fondle each other. Sitting positions have practical benefits in tight spaces as well; places like your tub, bathrooms, and cars.

MAY

It's a Digital World

The variety of ways you can use your hand and fingers to pleasure yourself are almost endless. Learning how you like to stroke, rub, or massage yourself will also make it easier for you to show a lover how to please you. Here are a couple of one-handed techniques to try:

+ **One-Finger Salute.** Rub your rosebud with your middle finger, side-to-side or in circles.

+ **Two-Finger Twiddle.** Massage your clitoris in a circular motion with your index and middle finger. Or take any two fingers and slide them up and down your inner labia on either side of your clitoris, stimulating the entire area.

+ **Two-Finger Roll.** Hold the shaft of your clitoris between your thumb and index or middle finger. Roll it between your fingers. Pull, pinch, squeeze, and release to your heart's content.

+ **Three-Finger Spread.** Use your index finger and ring finger to spread your outer labia while your middle finger rubs your clitoris.

+ **Count to Ten.** Draw the numbers one to ten on your vulva with one or two fingers. The number eight is especially nice: Glide your fingers from the top of your vulva down around your clitoris to your vaginal opening, around and up again.

+ **Three's Company.** Hold three or four fingers side-by-side and slide them up and down over your entire clitoral area, or vibrate them in any direction.

If you find direct stimulation too intense, try the surrounding areas, or pleasure yourself through your underwear, a bed sheet, or some other fabric. Again, experimentation is key when you're making love to Number One.

MAY

Can I Get a Hand Here?

The nice thing about one-handed work is that it leaves your other hand free to pleasure the rest of your body at the same time. While you're diddling your love button, tweak your nipples into hardness, rolling them between your fingers or massaging them in circles with your open palm. Stroke your derriere. Put a finger at the opening of your vagina and pretend it's your lover's penis, waiting to plunge inside.

You can also bring your other hand into the action down below. Use one hand to gently spread your outer labia, tightening the skin around your clitoris. Then stimulate yourself with your other hand using any technique you want. Tap your clitoris with your middle finger, imagining that it's your man's penis, or bat quickly with your index and middle finger. Stroke your exposed clitoris up and down.

You free hand doesn't have to hold still, of course. Use it to massage your vaginal lips while you pleasure yourself with your other hand. Pull lightly on your pubic hair. Stimulate the underside of your clitoris with the fingers of one hand as you rub the top with the other. Or hold your clit with the fingers of one hand as you rub circles over it with the palm or fingers of the other. Massage your perineum (the spot between your anus and vagina) with your fingertips, and then slide both hands up through the growing wetness of your vagina to your clitoris. Be voluptuous. Be creative.

MAY

Take a Seat

Spice up your love life by moving your trysts out of the bedroom. For this next lusty move, which is an expanded version of February 18th's tip, head to the living room. He sits on a couch or a comfortable (but firm) chair; you face away from him and lower yourself onto his waiting erection, your legs astride his and your feet planted firmly on the ground. If you put all your weight on him, his thrusting will be limited, but he will be free to fondle your breasts and clitoris. Put your hand over his and show him exactly what to do. Of course, he may already know from watching you masturbate (you do let him watch, don't you?) that this position allows him to achieve the same angle as your hands. If you've got strong thigh muscles, you can also hover a little bit above him, teasing the tip of his member until he can't help but pull you down onto him.

The Taoist pillow book *T'ung Hsüan Tzu* gives this position the delightful name The Goat and the Tree, evoking an animal in heat satisfying her desires against a phallic pole. You can certainly turn this position into a game. Sit on his lap while he's fully clothed and begin rocking back and forth. Suggest that you watch a porn video together while you're perched on his knee. Give him a private lap dance. See how long it is before your casual moves prompt more salacious activities.

MAY

Hump Day

So your hands are tired? Why not ride your pillow, a pile of sheets or even a bunched-up duvet? Take a little walking tour through your house and rub against whatever surface strikes your fancy: the bathroom sink, the back of a chair, your desk corner. Throw a towel over the padded arm of a chair or sofa, and have a seat with your legs spread. Gyrate against the arm until you're driving yourself crazy.

Transform laundry day from a chore into a pleasure by sitting on a corner of the washing machine during the spin cycle. Speaking of clothes, you can get them into the act, too. Pull your thong underwear tight against your clit and rub away, or buff yourself against the crotch of your jeans.

Look around your home. You'll discover a panoply of objects that can be drafted for self-pleasuring, from candles to the rubber handles of cooking utensils. Wash a cucumber, carrot, or zucchini and make it wear a condom. Just don't use anything that could break, make sure it's clean and smooth, and wash it well afterwards. After you've sated your appetite, of course.

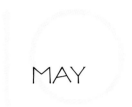

MAY

I'll Have the Combo Plate

Don't hesitate to get your entire body involved in your self-pleasuring sessions. Contract and relax your PC muscles (see January 7 and 8) rhythmically as you masturbate. Tighten your anus. Squeeze your thighs together or cross your legs. All of these moves tighten the area around your clit, sensitizing the entire region. Some women can come from this alone, opening up new worlds of possibilities for that boring work commute or weekly staff meeting.

Sure, it's important to focus on your clitoris, but don't neglect the rest of your genitals. Alternate between stimulating your love button and stroking your vagina or teasing the opening of your anus, which gets more sensitive as you become more aroused. In fact, while you're caressing your love button, see how it feels to penetrate your vagina—or even your anus—with a lubricated finger or two. You can simply dip your finger just inside, or thrust it in and out like your lover's penis. Try this move one-handed: Curl your hand so that you can massage your clitoris with your thumb as you relish the feeling of penetration.

You can also experiment with different positions. Pleasure yourself while sitting, standing, squatting, or kneeling. Lie on your stomach or side. Keep your legs open or closed, knees up or down. Mix it up!

MAY

Mother's Day Tips

Parenthood and a fulfilling sex life don't have to be mutually exclusive, but give yourself a break: It's okay if you're not going at it like rabid monkeys. My friend Anne, a consultant in her early forties with two adorable tykes, gives this advice to mothers with little ones: "Don't beat yourself up if you don't have as much sex as you used to. You just won't for a while, so relax. You *will* have fun sex again!"

Of course, the biggest battle faced by parents of young children is simple exhaustion. Having sex at the end of the day, after the kids are in bed and you're dead tired, may simply be impossible. Anne offers a creative solution: "Find a trusted sitter or family member to watch the kids, but instead of you and your mate going out, *stay home while the kids leave for the evening!* Reserve enough time with your sitter so that you can take a bath together (or let mom take one alone if that's what she needs), give each other massages, and then get busy. Because the kids' outing will probably have to happen during the day or early evening, you'll have more energy. It will feel like a vacation alone, and you'll have fun sex for the first time in ages. It's cheaper and more feasible than a hotel or spa getaway, but still lots of fun!"

Happy Mother's Day!

MAY

Position of the Week: Ananga Ranga Sitting Positions

The *Ananga Ranga* of late medieval India describes a variety of sitting positions, many of which seem more like positions for meditation than lovemaking. With Kama's Wheel, for example, the man keeps his legs outstretched as the woman lowers herself onto him. He keeps his arms straight on either side of her, supporting her shoulder blades in his hands, so that his limbs resemble the spokes of a wheel. In the Lotus Position, your lover keeps his legs crossed as you sit on his lap, your legs stretched out behind him. A variation called the Accomplishing Position calls for you to raise one leg slightly, changing the sensation for your vagina and his penis.

To achieve the nicely named Position of Equals, lean back so that your hands are resting on his shins, and stretch your legs around his body under his elbows, clasping your feet around his back. If you both lean back at the same time so that you can hold each other's feet, you're doing the Snake Trap. You probably won't get much stimulation in this position, but you can rock back and forth with each thrust. Look deep into his eyes, or use this opportunity to watch what's going on down below.

MAY

Give Him a Hand

You've spent much of this month learning to get a grip on yourself. Now, let's take a little detour to discuss fun ways to get a grip on him. Master the art of the perfect hand job, and he'll be putty in your hands.

So how do you get started, especially if he's still fully clothed? First get him warmed him up with lots of kissing and fondling. Now slide your hand down his chest and stomach to the rapidly growing bulge in his pants. Speaking of which, take those pants into account—if he's wearing loose slacks, you've got some room to play with, but if he's sporting tight jeans, you'll need to approach him a little more carefully. Don't just reach and grab, or you'll be rewarded for your efforts by a scream of pain. Instead, gently massage his erection through the fabric with a flattened hand.

By now, his manhood will be straining to be set free. It's your duty to liberate it, but be careful. Undo his belt buckle, open all the buttons, or unzip the zipper all the way. Slowly. You want to make sure you're free and clear before going in. Don't try to pull his member out through the flaps in the fly, instead pull down the elastic so his penis peeps out the top. This is a good time to ease his pants over his hips; you can certainly leave them pooling around his ankles if you want him to restrict his movements, so that he feels erotically imprisoned. Now it's time to get to work!

MAY

Wet His Whistle

In case you haven't noticed, your man's equipment doesn't come with its own lubricant. A few drops of pre-come isn't going to hack it. Some men may want you to stroke their penises dry, especially if they're uncircumcised (the foreskin can act as a natural lubricant); if so, you'll need to use a very gentle touch, because penis burn ain't fun.

The lubricant you use may depend on what's on your menu for later. Never—*never*—use any type of oil-based lubricant if you plan on having sex with a condom afterwards. Oils destroy latex. That includes massage oil, hand lotion, and any petroleum-based product like Vaseline. Instead, use a water- or silicone-based lube, and read the label if you're not sure.

If, however, a hand job is the only thing you've got planned, you have more options. Ask him what he likes. Lotions are popular, but they absorb into the skin, so you may want to keep a pretty pump bottle on your nightstand for touch-ups. Oils, including massage oils, stay slippery longer. You can even dip into the kitchen cupboard: vegetable, safflower, grapeseed, sunflower, and coconut oil can all work, but be careful about getting them inside you if you go on to have sex.

In a pinch, there's always your own saliva, which is a great option if you plan on augmenting your handwork with some oral action. If you think that dripping spit on his member is unladylike, simply get as much as you can onto your hand before you reach for his joystick.

MAY

Handwork: The Basics

So you've got his love wand out of his pants, and your hand is all lubed up and ready for action. (It's also clean and well-manicured, but you already know that.) What now? First, think about staging. If you're right-handed, lie or sit on his right side; if you're left-handed, position yourself on his left. You can also lie back and have him straddle your stomach as he kneels over you, giving you unfettered access. Or you can kneel between his legs as he lies back. Use your imagination: Kneel on the floor in front of him as he sits on a chair; sit while he stands in front of you; or wrap yourself around him from behind and reach around in front.

Now it's time to get a grip—the firmer, the better. As my good friend Kyle says, think of it as a baseball bat, not china. The most sensitive areas are the head; the rim around the bottom of the head; the ridge running along the underside; and the super-sensitive piece of skin on the underside that connects the head to the shaft. You can start by wrapping your fingers around his shaft with either your thumb or pinky resting against the rim, or by making a ring of your thumb and index finger.

No matter what position your hand is in, keep in contact with his member at all times, using a smooth, consistent motion. Ask him to show you how he pleasures himself; your fascinated gaze will be a huge turn-on. Put your hand over his as he strokes. Watch him during mutual masturbation sessions. When in doubt, ask!

MAY

Awakening the Second Chakra

In Tantra, the genital area is the seat of the second chakra, the energy center relating to our sexual urges and fantasies, creativity (and procreativity), and emotions. When this chakra is "open" and healthy, we experience stable, joyful emotions and self-acceptance, especially in areas concerning our sexuality. But when the second chakra is blocked by negative programming about sex, sexual abuse, or shame about sexuality, we experience a host of emotional and sexual difficulties. By awakening the deep feeling residing in our second chakra, we awaken our deeper capacity for pleasure.

Here's an exercise for awakening your second chakra adapted from one outlined by Tantric expert David Ramsdale, my co-author of *Red Hot Tantra*. Hold your hands in front of you, palms facing each other. Breathe deeply, and imagine you're holding a bright ball of energy. Move the ball down to the lowest part of your belly, and visualize it feeding your root chakra (see April 17). Now move the ball up into your womb, and color it orange. Imagine streams of energy, thick as honey, radiating out from the ball. Imagine these streams embracing your genitals and womb with healing orange light, and spreading to the sides of your body at the same level. Keep it there for about five minutes. (It's fine if your lover wants to pleasure you during this process.) Take the energy up through the other chakras, spending one or two minutes at each, or remain at the first two. When you've had enough, bring the energy back down and "ground" it by closing your palms together or pressing them against the wall.

Try practicing this exercise for one to three months, although you may experience results—including more blissful orgasms—much sooner.

MAY

Why Use a Vibrator? Reason #1: They're for Everyone!

One of the great things about using vibrators is that they are equal-opportunity sex toys. Vibrators don't discriminate against anyone because of gender, sexual orientation, weight, or race. They don't care if you're carrying a few extra pounds or don't feel like putting on your makeup that day. They don't need all your attention: A vibrator doesn't care if you have someone else in bed with you. Vibrators are simply there to help everyone feel good.

Men can have fun with vibrators as well, alone or with their partners. After all, men appreciate a variety of stimuli, just as women do, and a vibrator is another potential source of pleasure. Guys who feel wary about playing with something that looks like a penis can certainly enjoy the traditional massagers found in drugstores, as well as vibrating sleeves, cock rings, and anal toys.

If you have a disability, the intense stimulation offered by vibrators can help overcome reduced sensitivity. Pregnant women find that vibrators relieve soreness and help them achieve orgasms even in the late stages of pregnancy, when they might have trouble reaching their genitals. New moms report that a gentle massage with a battery-powered vibrator can calm crying babies. (Remember that scene in *Sex in the City* where Samantha puts a vibrator in the crib of Miranda's son to stop him from crying?)

Even if you have a "perfect sex life," vibrators can spice up your sexual routine. So if you have a vibrator, get creative with it. If you don't, keep an open mind!

Shop 'til You Pop

So you want to venture into the wonderful world of adult toys, but you don't know where to start? Don't worry if you've had some bad experiences with the useless novelties found in adult stores, or if you're a complete novice. These days, buying a good vibrator is easier than ever. First, do some research. The Good Vibrations Web site is a great place to start, as are books like Joani Blank's *Good Vibrations: The Complete Guide to Vibrators, Sex Toys 101,* or *Toygasms!* by Sadie Allison.

Once you know a little bit more about what you might like, visit a sex-positive adult store and ask the helpful sales staff for advice. The resources in books like *The Good Vibrations Guide to Sex* list numerous shopping outlets as well. Don't be embarrassed to call or email one of these specialty retailers. They've heard it all, and they're glad to help. If they aren't, try someplace else!

You can also buy vibrators in almost any drugstore, department store, and electronics store today—they're marketed as "massagers." (Manufacturers don't advertise these products' lustier benefits!)

Like shoes, you can find a vibrator to suit your every mood. You might find that one style suits you just fine, or you might acquire an entire toy chest of pleasure wands. The only requirement is a desire to have fun... lots of fun!

MAY

Position of the Week: For Crying Out Loud

The Crying Out Position of the *Ananga Ranga* is sure to provoke some moans of delight. Start in a sitting position, with your man sitting at the head of the bed, his back supported by lots of pillows. Slowly lower yourself onto him, letting him feel your delicious wetness inch by inch. Let him lift you slightly by slipping his hands under your legs so that your legs drape over his arms. This enables him to clasp you by the hips or buttocks and move you from side to side on his erect member. He can move you backward and forward, too; this variation is known as the Monkey Position. In Sheikh Nefzawi's *The Perfumed Garden*, this position is also called The Alternate Movement of Piercing, no doubt because instead of thrusting with his pelvis, your man moves you on his member.

Obviously, you need to need to have spent some serious time in the gym or yoga studio to do these positions as described in the ancient erotic texts. But although they seemed designed to be best enjoyed if your man is larger and stronger than you, equal-sized couples can enjoy them with some modification. For example, you can lean back and support yourself on your hands, and rock your pelvis in time with his movements. Or, instead of draping your legs over his arms, you can rest them on his upper thighs. Use the original position suggestion, and then get creative!

MAY

Talk Dirty to Me

Some people find "dirty talk" incredibly exciting. While you may need to tread lightly in this area, dirty language has incredible erotic power. Even the *promise* of dirty talk can start some lovers' engines. Just whisper "Do you mind if I talk dirty?" in your man's ear, as though whatever he's doing is causing you to throw all sense of propriety to the winds. Chances are he'll say "no," and you'll have full rein to unleash your Inner Porn Star—or your Inner R-Rated Star, as the case may be.

What do you say? For some people, a feverish "Fuck me, fuck me, fuck me" works just peachy. Repeat at will. If you don't feel comfortable with x-rated language, even saying "I want you inside me *now*" can be very sexy.

NOTE: This is not a license to chatter throughout the entire sex act. Some people like to focus as they approach an orgasm, and talk just distracts them. Like a spice, talk is best used as an accent. Those nonverbal cues, your "oohhs" and "aaahhhs," and "mmmms" will tell your lover everything he or she wants to know.

MAY

Gemini: The Twins

Were you or your man born between today and June 21? If so, you fall under the third sign of the zodiac: Gemini, symbolized by twins, and ruled by the planet Mercury. Astrologers consider Geminis to be vivacious, witty, and versatile, with highly developed intellects that need constant stimulation. You'll never have a dull moment with a Gemini, as they love lively conversation and new experiences, sexual or otherwise.

Whether you or your partner is a Gemini, remember that variety is the spice of a Gemini's life. Keep things fresh by organizing "spontaneous" sexual adventures: Perch on the edge of your washing machine and seduce him in the laundry room. Sit on his lap while you're wearing nothing underneath your long, flowing skirt. Master the art of the quickie. Surprise him with your lusty thoughts and deeds. Dazzle him with your sexual personae. Will he encounter a shy maiden or voluptuous vixen tonight? Only you know.

Keep him on his toes, so to speak, with lots of variety during the act of lovemaking itself. Start out in a sitting position, then push him back and mount him in a reverse cowgirl. If he's on top, take charge and roll over on top. Challenge him to see how many *Kama Sutra* positions you can accomplish in one session. Keep him guessing, and you'll both keep coming back for more.

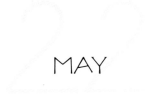

MAY

Lust: It's Even Better than Old Spice

In this very lusty month of May, let your inner strumpet burst forth. One way to do this is to occasionally relax your hygiene rules. This doesn't mean that you should go without showering for a week, it just means that you don't *always* have to be scrubbed clean before you jump between the sheets. Let him see and smell your sweaty body after your Saturday soccer game. The salty scent of *you* can act like a natural aphrodisiac. Plus, exercise raises your endorphin levels just like sex, so don't be in such a hurry to cool down after you work out. You're giving off the same aroma as you do during a passionate lovemaking session— and on some base, primal level, he senses it. Let nature work for you once in a while.

In a similar vein, don't be in such a hurry to change the bed linens. Sure, you can try dousing the sheets with some musky perfume, but why not let your own scents linger for a while? The smell of your partner will trigger the same chemical response you have when you're canoodling under the covers together. And as long as you keep yourself clean down there, your body's own lubricant is a fine aphrodisiac. Dip a finger into your own vaginal juices and give him a brief whiff by drawing a finger under his nose or placing it on his lips. He'll be in the mood immediately.

MAY

Straddle Him on the Sofa

The *Kama Sutra* and other erotic texts delight in portraying lovers cavorting in lush gardens, but you don't have to go outside to liven up your lovemaking. Just head to the living room. While your partner sits on your sofa, or a comfortable chair, sit on his lap with your knees up against his chest and your feet on either side of his hips. Lean back—if you're super-limber, stretch your arms all the way back to the floor like you're doing a backbend—and start thrusting. Open and close your legs and grasp him with your PC muscle to give him a variety of sensations that will get his juices flowing, or bend over the back of the couch to offer him entry from behind.

Got a rocking chair? Mount him while he's sitting there and rock back and forth together. You can brace your feet against the floor for added leverage. Just make sure it's a sturdy chair—you don't want it to collapse as you're singing your own erotic version of *Rock-a-Bye-Baby*.

And don't just think about seating when you're in the living room. Clear off the coffee table and lie on top of it with your hips at the edge. Chances are it will be just the right height for him to kneel in front of you and partake of the many delights your body offers.

MAY

When Heading South, Attitude Is Everything

The secret to giving great oral pleasure is to approach your task with gusto. This way, you're almost guaranteed success, because there is almost nothing a man loves more than a woman enthusiastically sucking his penis. Be honest: Don't you get off, just a little, in making him your sexual slave through your expert use of the oral arts?

Some people feel squeamish about oral sex because they're afraid that they or their partner will taste or smell bad, but if you both keep yourselves clean, there's nothing to worry about. You can always take a romantic bath or shower together before you get busy.

Some women also worry about gagging while performing oral sex. You can control your natural gag reflex not only through practice, but also by wrapping your saliva-moistened hand around your lover's penis, so you can control the depth of his thrusting. (Combining hand and mouth work enhances the pleasures of both activities, by the way.) Take him into your mouth as much as feels comfortable, and then relax your throat muscles. Exhale through your nose as you slide down his member. Speed up gradually, keep breathing, and don't hesitate to come up for air if you really need to.

In most men, wonderful genital kissing produces a desire to reciprocate either in kind or with crazy monkey sex. So show him that you really crave his member. Indulge your oral fixation. Be a tease. Have fun!

MAY

Bobbing Along

To give your man wonderful mouth work, pay close attention to his body language. If he starts moaning in crazed ecstasy when you do something, that's usually a pretty good sign. You could also simply ask him what he likes. Does he want you to concentrate on the head, the base, or a combination? Does he like firm pressure, or gentle? Does he want you to imitate a vacuum cleaner or flick your tongue like a butterfly? Or does he like the whole smorgasbord?

There's much more to mouth mastery than sucking. Attitude, for one. Kneel between his legs—there are other positions, but we'll get to those another day—and gaze at his manhood with the awe you bestow on your favorite ice cream. Form an "L" with each hand, and place them at the base of the shaft. Lick the sides of the shaft and the tip, then, putting your lips over your teeth (or keeping them loose like an "O"), slide the head inside your mouth and lick it like you would an ice cream cone.

What you do next will let him know right away that there's ecstasy in store. Relax your mouth, neck, and jaw, and take his entire penis into your mouth in one fell swoop and then pull back up, letting your lips pop over the ridge between his shaft and his tip. After this winning introduction, bob up and down, sucking gently. No Hoovers, please, because they'll throw off your rhythm. Make the most of your tongue until he begs for mercy.

MAY

Position of the Week: Frog Fashion

Many of the sitting positions described in erotic texts like *The Perfumed Garden* and the *Ananga Ranga* allow very little movement by either partner, so they seemed best designed for times when you want to take a break from more vigorous lovemaking.

For example, in the position described in *The Perfumed Garden* as Frog Fashion (and in the *Ananga Ranga* as the Paired Feet Position), your man sits with his legs apart, knees bent, as you lower yourself onto him. Then, you lean back onto some pillows or a cushion as you bend your knees and press your thighs together so that your knees meet at his chest. Keep your feet apart so that he can still penetrate you; hold onto your shins if necessary. If you're both really limber, you may even able to tuck your toes under his legs, which will push your heels back against your buttocks even further. The pressure of your thighs will constrict your vagina, producing wonderful sensations for both of you. Your man can then grasp your shoulders or upper arms to keep you close. Neither of you will be able to move very much, so put those Kegel exercises to good use!

Use sitting positions as an opportunity to deepen your intimacy. Look into each other's eyes, and focus on the sensation of his lingam in your wet yoni.

MAY

X Marks the Spot

The ancient love texts do depict some sitting positions that allow the woman to take a more active role. The position designated Pounding on the Spot in *The Perfumed Garden* is one of these. Have your man sit on the bed—he might want to prop himself against the headboard to support his back—as you sit astride his thighs and guide his penis into your aroused vagina. Put your arms around each other and cross your legs around his back. Using your thigh muscles, move up and down on him. If you've ever taken English-style horseback riding lessons, you'll know the move: It's like "posting" during the trot.

To drive him absolutely wild, tighten your PC muscle each time you slide down onto him. Enjoy the fact that with this position, you're in control of the rhythm and depth of penetration. You can bounce up and down on his lap, or slow things down to gentle thrusting. Meanwhile, he doesn't have to be passive. Guide his hands to your derriere: He can not only support you by your buttocks, but create some highly erotic sensations by spreading them and caressing your crease, anus, and perineum. Rock your pelvis so your clitoris rubs against his pubic bone. As you pound on his hot spot, you may just rediscover yours!

MAY

Vibe Shopping Guide

On May 18, we gave you some ideas on where to shop for a vibrator. Now it's time to talk about *how*. Here's a checklist you may want to copy and carry in your purse next time you go shopping:

+ **Purpose.** What do you want to stimulate? Your clitoris? Vagina? G-spot? Anus? All of the above? Will you use your vibe with a partner, or alone?

+ **Portability.** Is your vibrator going to stay in your bedroom, or will it accompany you on the road? If it's the latter, look for smaller, battery-operated or rechargeable electric vibes.

+ **Noise.** Do you care if the neighbors hear? If so, your best bets are virtually silent coil-operated electric vibes. Battery-operated and wand vibrators tend to be louder.

+ **Intensity.** Do you want gentle or strong vibrations? A general rule: The smaller the battery, the less the vibration.

+ **Price.** A vibrator will run you anywhere from $10 to $80 or more, but think of it as an investment, and remember that you get what you pay for. An electric vibrator from a brand-name manufacturer will last you for years.

+ **Shape.** Vibrators these days come in a truly mind-boggling assortment of shapes and styles. Do you want something realistic or smooth?

+ **Color.** Yes, color. Do you prefer flesh tones? Or do you want to get more festive with metallic, glow-in-the-dark, or jewel-toned toys?

If you think about these aspects before you buy, you'll have any easier time wading through the variety of vibrators out there. You'll also ask better questions of the sales staff. Best of all, you'll be happier with your purchase when you get it home!

MAY

First Time With a Vibe?

So you've been shopping, you've brought your new vibrator home (or it's arrived in the mail), and it's unwrapped and ready to go. What now?

Whether it's your first time with a vibrator or you simply want to get the most out of it, remember to take your time. Run your vibrator all over your body, from your shoulders to your feet. Get in whatever position you find most comfortable; you can always experiment. When you're ready, touch your genitals with the vibrator. You can always press it through your underwear or a cloth if you find direct genital stimulation too intense at first. You can either stroke yourself, or hold the vibrator against one spot. If your vibrator has more than one speed, try different speeds to see how it feels.

Test the vibrator on different places. Caress your clitoris or the clitoral hood. Press it against your mons, the fleshy mound that covers your pubic bone. Run it up and down your inner labia, and circle your vaginal opening. You can, of course, insert your vibrator into your aroused vagina, but remember that most of the nerve endings are concentrated in the entrance and lower third of the vagina, so most sensations will be near the opening. You'll probably need direct clitoral stimulation to climax, but everyone's different. And if you don't come the first time you use your vibrator, don't worry. You're just getting to know each other!

MAY

Toy Tips

As you'll soon discover (if you haven't already), the ways to use a vibrator are limited only by your imagination. Women can use vibrators for clitoral and vaginal stimulation; men can enjoy pleasuring their penis and testicles; and both sexes can relish in anal play and all-over skin massage. Here are ways to get the most pleasure from your pleasure toys:

+ **Get in the mood.** Watch pornos, read erotica, or fantasize—whatever gets your juices flowing.

+ **Experiment with body parts.** Try out the vibrator on different parts of your genitals and body.

+ **Experiment with positions.** Stimulate yourself lying on your back, side, or stomach.

+ **Try indirect pressure.** Put a piece of clothing, your hand, or a sheet between you and the vibrator to diffuse the sensations.

+ **Change the pressure and speed.** Start with light pressure and work up to steady, direct stimulation. Keep the speed low or turn it up several notches.

+ **Be a tease.** Start and stop. Turn off your vibrator for a while. Stimulate yourself in other ways, and then go back to where you were.

+ **Don't psych yourself out.** If you don't come, you don't come.

You'll also want to take good care of your beloved toy. It may sound obvious, but if you've got a battery-powered model, keep spare batteries on hand. Stock a back-up of your favorite vibe. There are few things more disappointing than having your vibrator conk out during a hot self-pleasuring session!

MAY

More Fun in the Great Outdoors

Hopefully you've found lots of ways this month to give full rein to your lustier urges. We started the month with some tips for an *al fresco* picnic to celebrate May Day. As May draws to a close, let's talk about some other ways to enjoy the intensely pleasurable experience of outdoor lovemaking.

If your garden or backyard guarantees absolute privacy, there's no reason why you can't enjoy your lusty picnic close to home. A backyard swing can be loads of fun. No backyard? Be creative: One romantic swain surprised his girlfriend by inviting her to meet him on the roof of their apartment building, where he was waiting in a child's wading pool filled with water, a bottle of champagne by his side. Who knows if they made it back downstairs on that warm summer night!

The great outdoors offers numerous options for lust. Who hasn't dreamed of making love on a beach (on a large blanket or towel, of course) accompanied by the sound of the waves? On a park bench, you can wriggle gently on his lap while wearing a long skirt and no underwear (penetration optional). Going on a hike in the woods? Face a tree, leaning against it, and have him bend his knees so he can enter you from behind and below while holding your hips to steady you. Camping? Make love under the stars, or find a sun-warmed boulder creekside. Afterwards, cool yourselves down in the flowing water, and imagine yourselves as Adam and Eve.

CHAPTER SIX

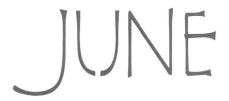

"I have embraced the summer dawn."
—Arthur Rimbaud (1854-1891), French poet,
from Illuminations, *"Aube"*

Get ready to embrace every summer dawn—erotically. June seems to be a month custom-designed to honor women. Historians believe that the ancient Romans named June after Juno, queen of the gods and protector of women. So this month, embrace your womanhood and express your creativity in your love-making, whether you're with a partner or by yourself. June 21 marks the summer solstice, so this month's tips will help you and your man take pleasure in each other's bodies during those long, lusty summer days and nights.

The Victorians gave each other this month's birth flower, *honeysuckle*, to represent generous and devoted affection. Keep vases of this sweet-smelling flower—as well as June's other birth flower, the *rose*, which has long been a symbol of love—around your home to remind yourself to openly express your affection not only to your loved ones but to yourself.

June's birthstone, the *pearl*, has a long and romantic history. The ancient Greeks believed that pearls were the hardened tears of joy that Venus, the goddess of love, shook from her eyes as she was born from the sea. Treat yourself to one piece of pearl jewelry (it doesn't have to be expensive!) to remind yourself that the spirit of Aphrodite lives within each of us.

JUNE

If You Can't Stand the Heat…

Get out of the bedroom, and *into* the kitchen! We all know that the kitchen is where everyone hangs out during a party. Why not make it the gathering place for your own private festivities? The kitchen counter makes a perfect surface for some delicious nooky. Instead of asking him to do the dishes, ask him to do you!

Perch on the edge of the counter with him standing in front of you, and wrap your legs around his waist. From this position, he can plunge into you without having to support your weight, leaving both his hands free to play with your beautiful breasts. Guide his thumb down to your clit as he pounds away, and you'll get some extra-tasty stimulation. Sitting on a horizontal surface like this is a nice way to transition to and from some of the standing positions we'll be talking about later in the month. Plus, if you're near the sink, you can run some water over your hands to cool yourselves down as thing heat up.

The counter and sink aren't the only places for kitchen sex play. Push him up against the refrigerator and ravish him. Or open it up and enjoy the contrast of cool air on your lust-inflamed body, as Colleen, a thirty-two-year-old artist, suggests: "I'll be doing something as simple as opening the fridge to get a drink when my guy will come up behind me and whisper something sweet, then something wonderfully nasty, while pressing his body against my back. He lets his hands wander everywhere until they reach major erogenous zones. By then I'm nearly falling into the cool refrigerator while my body explodes with heat." Is it getting hot in here?

HISTORICAL NOTE: Today is the birthday of film actress and sex icon Marilyn Monroe (1926-62).

JUNE

Position of the Week: Supported and Suspended Congress

Built in the tenth century A.D., the erotic temples of Khajuarho, India, are adorned with stunningly beautiful sculptures depicting explicit sexual acts. Many of the couples portrayed are shown in standing positions described in the *Kama Sutra*, the *Ananga Ranga*, and other ancient erotic texts. So surprise him by showing him your knowledge of ancient art, and seduce him standing up!

Standing positions can be extremely exciting for quickies (especially outdoors), or when passion simply overwhelms you before you can make it to the bed. Brace yourselves against each other or a wall to engage in what the *Kama Sutra* calls The Supported Congress. Wrap one of your legs around him to spread your thighs so that he can penetrate you more deeply (he can hold your thigh to give him more control as he thrusts). If he stands with his feet slightly parted, he'll be able to balance better.

If you really get carried away—and your man is pretty strong—have him lean against a wall or tree and wrap your arms around his neck as he lifts you onto him by holding your thighs or derriere. He can join his hands under your butt to give you more support as you push against the wall with your feet. This is The Suspended Congress position. You may not be able to maintain it very long—and make sure he doesn't drop you, or he could hurt his member—but you'll have fun trying!

HISTORICAL NOTE: Today is the birthday of Comte Donatien Alphonse François de Sade (1740-1814), the French novelist, playwright, and philosopher known by his title, the Marquis de Sade. The term *sadism*, used to describe the practice of getting sexual gratification from inflicting pain on others, derives from his name. Rent the movie *Quills* to find out more.

JUNE

Positions for Mouth Work (His)

When it's your turn to get some oral treats from your guy, there are several things you can do to make it more fun for both of you. The first is to try out different positions. For example, try propping a pillow or two under your butt, and one under his chest (it makes it more comfortable for your guy and gives him easier access). While you're at it, put a pillow under your head, too, so you can watch. No sense missing any of the action! Other variations:

✦ Sit on the edge of the bed or a chair and lean back while he kneels on the floor before you.

✦ Stand with your legs spread wide while he comes at you from underneath. Again, you may need something to hold onto in case your knees buckle!

✦ Get on all fours while he approaches you from behind. This definitely brings out the animal in some people. However, make sure he doesn't go back to your vulva if he indulges in any anal-oral play.

✦ To give his neck a break, move so that your man is approaching you from the side. You can both lie on your sides, too, with his head between your legs, resting on your thigh.

Not only is it sexy to change things around every so often, but it also keeps everyone's arms and legs from falling asleep. After all, there's nothing worse than a case of cunnilingus cramp.

HISTORICAL NOTE: On this day in 1937, the Duke of Windsor married American divorcee Wallis Warfield Simpson, for whom he had abdicated the throne of England the year before.

JUNE

Straddle Him

Lying on your back while your lover pleasures you orally might be the most comfortable position for you, but here's another interesting position for you to use when you want him to explore you with his mouth.

Have him lie on his back while you straddle his shoulders, kneeling on either side of him. Hold onto the headboard if necessary, lowering yourself onto him just enough so that he can take your clitoris in his mouth. You can also face towards his feet. To make it more comfortable for him, he might want to put a pillow or two under his head.

This position lets you control the pressure of your pleasure zone as his probing tongue explores your wetness. You can hold still, or rock back and forth. While you might not want to actually sit on his face—you don't want to smother the poor boy—you might be able to vibrate against his mouth, nose, and chin as you get closer to experiencing an orgasm. From this position, he'll also have a great view of the expressions of passion taking over your face, and he can fondle your derriere, tease your vaginal opening or anus with his fingers, or play with himself.

HISTORICAL NOTE: Today is the birthday of Josephine Baker (1906-75), the American singer and dancer whose revealing costumes and exotic routines—she performed once wearing nothing but a feather skirt—sent Parisian audiences into a frenzy. After fleeing the racism of the United States, she became a sensation in Europe.

JUNE

Positions for Mouth Work (Hers)

Just as you can position yourself for a better connection between his mouth and your cavern of love, so can you arrange yourself to delight his member in a variety of ways. Having him lie on his back while you lie or kneel between his legs is a common way to deliver oral action, but show him that you're a creative gal. Roll him gently onto his side and slide down the bed so that your face is even with his penis. In this position, he'll be able to thrust, and you'll get a break. Put a pillow below your head for even more support.

It may be a stereotype, but guys do get a thrill from standing or kneeling while a woman gives them head. Depending on your heights, you can worship at the altar of his erection in a number of ways. Kneel on the floor while he stands; have him kneel on the bed while you kneel on the floor; or have him kneel on the bed or floor while you sit in front of him, your legs wrapped around his thighs.

Another exciting position for him is when you lie on your back with him above you. You can either slide down the bed until you reach his member, or he can move up. He supports himself on his arms or the headboard while thrusting gently into your mouth. You may need to control his movements with your hands so he doesn't get carried away and thrust too deeply, but if not, busy your hands with his testes, perineum, and butt. The technical term for this practice is *irrumation*. Now, there's a cocktail party fact for you!

JUNE

A Helping Hand

You've got the lube, and you're in a comfortable position to give him manual pleasures. Now what? Ideally, you've watched how he masturbates, but it never hurts to surprise him with some variations.

First, master the basic stroke. Assuming you're lying side-by-side, grasp his member with your thumb at the top, and your pinky at the base. Put your other hand flat at the base of his penis, your fingers flat against his groin, your thumb wrapped around the base, and press gently. Your index finger and thumb should form a sort of "L." This increases the sensation to his member and keeps it stiff and steady as you play with it.

Now, slowly glide your grasping hand up toward the head until you're barely holding the tip, then slide back down the shaft. Start off slow and then speed up; gauge his reaction to see what speed to use. He may want you to stroke him fast with lots of pressure and lots of lube (just don't overdo it, or he won't feel anything), or he may just want to lay back and enjoy it slow, in which case you'll need less lube. As you pick up speed, you can remove your other hand from the base and stroke or cup his testicles. They'll like the attention, and so will he.

JUNE

Up, Over, and Down

Here's a manual technique that will drive your man wild. Again, press one hand against the base of his member. This time, when you grip him with your other hand, start so that your forefinger and thumb are at the bottom and your pinky is at the top, near the ridge. (The back of your hand will be facing you.)

Glide up to the top, but when you reach it, instead of going back down the way you came, twist over the head and caress it with your palm and fingers in a swiveling motion—almost like you were trying to screw in a light bulb with an open hand. You can even roll the head around in your palm. Whatever you do, don't let your hand lose contact with his staff. Then come down the other side, pinky finger first.

You can either repeat this up-and-over-and-down stroke with the same hand, or bring your other hand fluidly into play, alternating hands. This may sound complicated, but with a little practice, you'll soon get into the groove, and he'll be singing for joy.

JUNE

Let Him Take a Look

Many otherwise lusty women get a bad case of shyness when it comes to letting their man watch them masturbate. Get over it. Men are visual creatures, and the vast majority of them *love* to watch a woman pleasure herself. They *dream* about it. (Otherwise, it wouldn't be such a prominent activity in X-rated movies.) So give him a private show. Let him see you loving your body and your sexuality. Let him see the stages of your desire, arousal, and reaching an orgasm: How your chest flushes, how your breath quickens, how your muscles stiffen right before you climax, how your back arches as you lose control. When he sees how wet and horny you get, it'll be "Ladies first" from there on out.

If you're afraid that by letting him see you masturbate that he'll think he doesn't please you enough, well, heck, maybe he needs to learn a thing or two. Although men want to believe that their incredible sexual prowess is enough to send you into a frenzy, most of them are secretly flummoxed about what to do to achieve this, especially when they realize that (surprise!) every woman is different. What a relief for him to see exactly what pressure, stroking, and speed you need. Another way to approach it is that he just gets you so darn hot you can't keep your hands off yourself.

You can, of course, turn the show into a game. Forbid him to touch you, or tie him to the bed or a chair and force him to watch you make yourself come. He'll be begging to join the fun.

JUNE

Position of the Week: Belly to Belly

The Perfumed Garden by Sheikh Nefzawi describes two sensual standing positions. The first, Belly to Belly, is very similar to The Supported Congress of the *Kama Sutra*—you stand facing each other—except that you don't need to be leaning against a wall, and Nefzawi also suggests that your man extend one foot slightly forward. If he's taller than you, simply have him bend his knees while you stand on tiptoe. You won't be able to stay like this very long, but it will be a nice way to transition to horizontal or sitting positions.

What distinguishes this position is the detailed instructions the author gives for prolonging the excitement of penetration. Here, he suggests a move called The Bucket in the Well:

> *"The man and woman join in close embrace after the introduction. Then he gives a push, and withdraws a little; the woman follows him with a push, and also retires. So they continue their alternate movement, keeping proper time. Placing foot against foot, and hand against hand, they keep up the motion of a bucket in a well."*

Whether you're attempting a standing position or not, a technique like this can be an extremely exciting way to enhance your lovemaking. He doesn't even have to know you're doing it, but he'll definitely appreciate it.

JUNE

Plug in, Turn on

As you've seen, vibrators come in a dazzling array of sizes and shapes. Electric vibrators that plug into a standard 110-volt outlet are probably the most common type, simply because they're not marketed as sex toys but as "personal massagers," which means you can find them in many department and electronics stores. (Look for them among beauty care products.) Ironically, because they're *not* marketed for sexual purposes, you may have a harder time finding them in adult toy stores.

Electric vibrators usually offer a few different speeds or a rheostat (a dimmer switch, basically), allowing you to experiment with different pressures and speeds. Note that electric massagers often deliver quite powerful vibrations, which makes them great for all-over body massage but they're sometimes too intense for genital stimulation. If that's the case, try your electric vibe through clothes or fabric.

The good news is that since electric vibrators are made by brand-name manufacturers like Hitachi and Panasonic, they're made well and often come with one-year warranties. If you find one you like, it will be yours for years (unlike some boyfriends), and you don't have to worry about the batteries running out at inopportune moments. Many also come with attachments, allowing you to accessorize to your heart's content.

JUNE

Just Wave Your Magic Wand

Just like the name implies, electric wand vibrators look very much like a magic wand—and certainly can produce sensations that are nothing short of miraculous. Typically about a foot long, they feature a hard plastic handle and round, tennis-ball-sized rubber or acrylic head at one end. When you see one, you'll realize that it's designed specifically for external massage and not for penetration. The best-known electric vibrator is the Hitachi Magic Wand.

Because wand vibrators can deliver such intense vibrations, start out by pressing it through fabric—like a towel or piece of clothing—or near the clitoris rather than directly on it. The head will diffuse the sensations to the surrounding regions. In any case, start out slow (the fast speeds can be too intense in the beginning), and work yourself up to full-force, toe-curling climaxes. You can also vary your position when using a wand vibrator. Lie on top of it, grip it between your legs while you lie on your side, or prop it up on a pillow and lean forward on your knees.

Wand vibrators can also easily be incorporated into partner action. Hold the vibrator against the back of your hand as you grasp his member. If he can handle more intense stimulation, run it along the base of his penis or the shaft. You can also place it between you when he's on top; as you rub the wand on your clit, not only will he get stimulation to the base of his penis, but he'll also feel the vibrations inside your vagina. Don't be surprised if he wants you to wave your magic wand again and again.

JUNE

More Fun with Your Wand

The varieties of ways to use a wand vibrator are almost endless. Start by massaging it gently against your inner thighs. Then move to your outer and inner labia with long, slow strokes. As you move closer to your clit, you can buffer the sensations by putting three fingers together over your love bud, and pressing on the back of your fingers with the wand. Or be a tease: Raise the vibrator away from your body, pause and resume your lusty ministrations.

Are you ready for some direct stimulation of your rosebud? Slowly circle your wand around and over the tip of your clitoris. Stroke up and down. Tap it lightly against yourself. Press it firmly and gradually turn up the intensity until your entire body throbs with pleasure. Vibrate the wand against your clit as you slip your fingers around your wet opening and then deep inside yourself. See how it feels to press against your G-spot as you hold the vibrator against the part of the hand that's still outside.

Let your lover get some of the action, too. Show him how you like him to wield the vibrating staff, or have him cup one hand around the head of the buzzing vibrator, and then cradle that hand with the other. By extending two fingers of his outside hand, he's just turned it into a handy-dandy vibrating attachment with which to tease your clitoris, vagina, and G-spot into bliss.

JUNE

Self-Loving Reason #6: It's a Great Stress Reliever!

Stress is a fact of life. We may get stressed because of specific events, or as the result of general yuckiness in our lives—poor health, loneliness, or bad bosses. Unfortunately, high levels of stress can be toxic to your physical or emotional selves. You can manage your stress level in many ways, but in masturbation, you literally have a stress reliever right in the palm of your hand.

First, sexual arousal increases blood flow throughout your body, increasing your energy and dispelling the sluggishness that tends to be a stress byproduct. What's more, the intense, rhythmic muscular contractions produced by orgasm release built-up tension and send waves of endorphins—the body's natural painkillers—through the body. In fact, an orgasm is really the body's version of an oft-prescribed stress-reduction technique called *progressive muscle relaxation*, where you clench and release every muscle in your body.

You can experience the stress-relieving benefits of orgasms through lovemaking with your sweetie, but self-pleasuring is available to you anytime, anywhere. It isn't dependent on your loved one being in the mood—or being there at all—which can come in handy when you're on the road or between partners. No matter what your situation, masturbation can soothe away tension and anxiety like a good massage or a hot bath. Bad work week? Pesky boss? Demanding kids? Don't worry: Relief is at the tip of your fingers!

JUNE

Get Creative with Your Tunnel of Love

Sure, most women need direct clitoral stimulation in order to climax, but don't neglect your vagina during your self-loving sessions. Exploring its silky depths might get you warmed up for clit play or give your nubbin a break if you don't want to come just yet. Remember, most of the nerve endings are packed in the outer third of your vagina, so a little goes a long way. Dip one or two fingers inside and press upward. Swish around your vaginal canal in glorious circles, as though you were mixing up a delicious batter. If you curl your hand, you may even be able to massage your clit with your knuckles. Or bring the fingers of the other hand into play: With two fingers inside your vagina, press down on your clitoris and knead the tissues in between.

Another interesting technique is to lay your entire hand over your vulva, dipping your middle finger just inside your vagina and undulating your hand over your mons and clitoris like a teasing lover.

See what happens if you play with the skin around your vulva. Any time you pull it taut, you heighten the sensation on your clitoris and vaginal opening. Pull the skin of your pubic mound up toward your stomach, then slip your fingers in and out. Or spread your outer lips with your fingers and massage the inner ones with your thumb.

Any time you're exploring your vaginal depths is a great opportunity to flex your love muscle. Practice your Kegels during this kind of play, and you'll get a good idea of how incredible this move will feel for your partner.

JUNE

Sensual Shower Meditation

If you've got a handheld showerhead with a hose attachment, you've got a world of aquatic pleasure in store. Point the flow at your clitoris and vulva, and adjust the temperature and pressure as necessary. If your showerhead has a massager with various settings—from steady flow to a pulsing stream—play with the different settings. Put one foot on the side of the tub to keep your balance, and hold on! You may very well have a mystical experience, as my friend Connie relates:

"I've found a way to meditate and masturbate at the same time during my morning shower. I turn the shower massager on pulsate and place that drumbeat against my vulva. I begin by picturing two tongues of blinding yellow-white light twirling around my clitoris and engorging it with gentle, nurturing love. Then I move the light up into my vagina and throughout my womb, and let it fill every organ, cell, and tissue in my body with love. As I achieve an orgasm, I imagine this light coming out my nipples, mouth, and ears, blinding me.

"I keep my hand over my mound to coax the smaller, slowly receding climaxes until they subside along with the light. I'm left with a feeling of peace as I turn off the water, return the massager to its hook and step out of the shower, ready to start my day!"

JUNE

Position of the Week: Driving the Peg Home

The wonderful thing about the ancient erotic texts is their wildly creative descriptions of lovemaking—descriptions that seem to demonstrate a real artistic appreciation for the beauty and excitement of the sexual act. Take the *Perfumed Garden's* second standing position, Driving the Peg Home. As with The Supported Congress, your ardent suitor lifts you up onto him as you wrap your legs and arms around him, only this time he holds you with your back against the wall. His member plunges into you like a peg being driven into a wall—hence the name.

Positions like these remind of us those moments when we feel crazy lust for the object of our affections. If you can't wait until you get home, or simply can't make it to the bed, why not have him take you where you are—against a tree, in a hallway, or in a coat closet at a crowded party? As summer heats up, there's no reason you can't generate some heat as well.

NOTE: As thrilling as this position is, please don't try it unless your man is strong enough to support you. If he drops you while he's still inside you, he could seriously injure himself (see March 18). We want safe sex to be just that.

JUNE

Use Him for Your Pleasure

You know how fascinated your man is with his own member? He'll think it's incredibly thrilling if *you* find it just as enthralling. Use his penis—and the rest of his body—for your own pleasure. Many men find nothing sexier. One guy relayed that he tells his girlfriend to use him as her own personal sex toy, and he gets incredibly aroused when she happily obliges. Why? Simple. He gets turned on when you get turned on, and when it's *his own body* that's turning you on, it's a real boost to his masculinity.

So when your man tells you that he wants you to be selfish in bed, he doesn't mean he wants you to be a jerk: He means that he wants you to enjoy yourself to hilt. He wants you to forget about pleasing him like the good little girl you were trained to be, and focus instead on getting yourself off like the lusty sex goddess you deserve to be. There's nothing he likes to see more than your body in the throes of passion, so show your guy that his body is an instrument to your ecstasy. Rub his penis all over your body—your neck, your breasts, your belly, your thighs. Massage it against your clitoris, like you would a dildo or vibrator. Do whatever you need to do to achieve an orgasm. Think "Ladies first," and mean it.

It's kind of a Zen thing. If once in a while you *don't* concern yourself with his pleasure—only your own—you're almost guaranteed to pleasure him all the more.

JUNE

Pregnancy and Sex

When you're pregnant, your body morphs into something completely new. You may find that your libido does a nosedive, particularly during the first trimester, or conversely, that soaring hormones, freedom from birth control, and pride in your body's creativity may turn you into a virtual sex monster. During the second trimester in particular, the increased blood flow to your genitals will swell your erectile tissues; meanwhile, higher levels of estrogen mean more vaginal lubrication. At this stage, you may experience higher levels of arousal and stronger orgasms.

Whatever your experience, be flexible with your fluctuating desire levels (as well as your partner's). Be open to trying out new techniques and methods of stimulation. Also, be aware that orgasms and intercourse are perfectly safe during a normal, healthy pregnancy. Exceptions are if you're at risk for premature labor, have a history of miscarriage, or have other medical conditions. Ask your doctor.

As your due date nears, pamper yourself. Let your hubby know—in a loving way—how much you would appreciate a little extra TLC. My friend Talila, a writer, offers a couple of tips for the guys. "Speaking as a pregnant woman in her ninth month, I can tell you that pampering has been key to our relationship recently. A shoulder rub or a foot massage instantly puts me in a good mood—even though I'm chronically uncomfortable these days. Flattery also helps. Even though the scale and the mirror remind me of my weight gain each day, my husband's frequent compliments are enormously reassuring. Sincere comments like 'You're the most beautiful pregnant woman' or 'Your skin is so radiant' win him the big points."

Ask him for what you need. You just might get it!

JUNE

Awakening the Third Chakra

You know when someone says they had a "gut feeling" about something? Tantrists believe it's emanating from their third, or belly, chakra, the energy center from which our emotions originate. Our sense of personal power resides in our upper belly (or solar plexus), while our sexual energy is reflected in our lower belly. Unexpressed emotions such as love, anger, or fear stick in our guts, blocking this chakra. Unfortunately, if you repress your emotions, chances are that you'll repress your sexuality as well. After all, if you construct a suit of armor to protect your belly, how can your sexual passion have free rein?

As a specific exercise, try meditating for at least ten minutes to see what emotions come up. Observe your feelings, but don't judge. If you feel angry, be aware of that fact. Don't try to analyze it. Afterwards, you might want to jot some notes down in your journal, but for these ten minutes, simply sit quietly and see what happens. Later, if it feels safe, ask your sweetie to gently massage your abdomen, working from the center out, and then down toward your pubic bone. If you can stop "protecting" your belly, you'll open yourself up to the sexual fire waiting inside.

JUNE

Hand Work When You're Going South

When you're giving your fella fellatio, there's no need to let your mouth do all the work. Let your hand act as an extension of your mouth. Make a ring with your index finger and thumb (like you're giving the okay sign), or with your entire hand, and place it at the base of his shaft. Keep it close to your lips, but as you bob up with your head, slide your fingers down with a tight grip. He'll feel like he's getting a blowjob and a hand job at the same time, and it will drive him nuts (in a good way).

For variety, you can also slide your hand up along with your mouth; let his penis peek up through your index and middle finger, and then slide back down. When you come up, his wand goes back through the ring. The tighter you keep your fingers and mouth, the better it should feel to him—but ask, just to be sure. You can also twist your hand slightly as you go.

Another way to use your hands while you're going down on him is by making a ring around the base of the shaft—about an inch from the bottom—and pulling down. This will pull the skin of his penis taut, which increases the sensitivity of the head. It will also make him hard quicker—and possibly give him an orgasm faster—which in some situations (an airplane bathroom, a pre-work quickie, your jaws are tired) can be kind of handy. So to speak.

JUNE

Extended Loving Hours on the Summer Solstice

Today marks the summer solstice, the longest day of the year, so take advantage of the extended daylight hours by using the following technique to make your lovemaking last and last. The key is to stimulate him as long as possible, because the longer his arousal, the more intense his orgasm. To ensure his cooperation, you may want to give him a brief idea of what you're about to do. (You may also want to tie him down and drive him crazy, but that's your call.)

If you're going down on him or giving him a hand job, you can easily control the pace. Watch him carefully for signs that his orgasm is getting close: His muscles may stiffen, his breath may come faster, or his chest may flush. Before he gets to the point of no return, stop what you're doing for at least ten seconds. If you're making love, you can slow and then stop your own thrusts; ask him to slow down; or simply let him slip out of you.

Once he's calmed down, re-start what you were doing—or try something new—until he's close to coming again. Then stop for a second time. If you want to start and stop again, you can, but don't stop more than three or four times, or he may not be able to climax at all. When you want him to come at last, intensify your movements: Stroke or suck him faster, or if he's inside you, thrust harder, clutch him with your PC muscles, and caress him all over. When he finally climaxes, he'll have one of the most incredible, shuddering orgasms of his life.

Note that the same technique works for you, so if you practice these techniques together, you'll increase your orgasm intensity tenfold.

JUNE

Cancer: The Crab

If you or your lover were born between June 22 and July 22, you fall under the water sign of Cancer, symbolized by a crab. Cancerians are thought to be home-loving, nurturing, sensitive, and artistic people who are deeply aware not only of their own feelings and emotions but others' emotions as well. Appeal to your Cancerian lover's need to be nurtured (and to nurture you in return) by suggesting that you prepare a romantic, candlelit meal together, ideally featuring your favorite comfort foods. Start your foreplay in the kitchen. As you're preparing the meal, give each other little tastes from the dish, washed down by sips of a nice wine. Build your anticipation by touching each other frequently as you're cooking. Cozy up to him from behind as he's stirring the soup. Give his butt a quick squeeze on your way to the refrigerator.

After your meal, move into the bedroom for dessert. Remembering that Cancerians are romantic sensualists, give him an opportunity to express his voluptuous sensuality—or for you to express yours—by engaging in some erotic role play. Tell him that you're going to play a little game called Sultan and Harem Girl—or Sultaness and Harem Boy, depending on your mood. The idea is that for one night, one person will administer to the other's every sexual need. Start with an erotic massage, and then put yourself at his disposal. If you're the one in charge, here's your chance to vocalize your every sexual whim! Whether you fall under the sign of Cancer or not, this game is guaranteed to coax even the shyest lover out of his or her shell.

JUNE

"Love looks not with the eyes, but with the mind;
And therefore is wing'd Cupid painted blind."
—*William Shakespeare (1564-1616), A Midsummer Night's Dream.*

Midsummer's Eve Madness

Throughout Europe, people have observed Midsummer's Eve with joyous celebrations, dancing, and bonfires at festivals that are believed to be continuances of Teutonic pagan fertility rites. In Sweden and Finland, Midsummer's Eve festivals are the largest of the year, and are noted not only for their tradition of raising and dancing around a somewhat phallic maypole, but also for their happy, drunken revelry.

You don't have to get drunk to observe your own private Midsummer's Eve festival, but you do have to act a little pagan. Fill your living room with candlelight and spread a blanket on the floor. Open a bottle of your favorite wine or champagne, and then prepare an indulgent feast. There are only three rules: 1) no utensils; 2) no clothes; 3) no feeding yourself. Feeding each other with your fingers is not only nurturing but highly erotic as well. For appetizers, choose finger foods like chilled asparagus spears, baby carrots, or olives. Your main course can include treats like chicken wings, tiny red roasted potatoes or green beans. For dessert, feed each other decadent chocolate truffles or juicy in-season berries like strawberries, cherries, or blueberries. Dip the fruit in whipped cream.

Don't worry about making a mess. Savor each bite, and have fun licking the juices off each other. Indulge your oral fixation with tastes of food—and then with tastes of each other. End your Midsummer's Eve celebration with a dance. Whether you're horizontal or vertical is your choice.

HISTORICAL NOTE: Today is the birthday of Dr. Alfred Kinsey (1894-1956), American sexologist and author of *Sexual Behavior in the Human Male.*

JUNE

Position of the Week: The Congress of a Cow

Comparing a sexual position to a beast might seem somewhat unromantic to our twenty-first-century minds, but the ancients took great inspiration from the animal kingdom. The Congress of a Cow is a challenging *Kama Sutra* position that combines a standing position with rear entry. Start with him standing behind you and lean forward, feet apart, until your hands are touching the floor. (You can always put your hands on the bed if you're not as limber, or if you start to get a head rush.) Steady yourself as he enters you from behind.

By holding your hips and waist, he can pull you against him in time with his thrusts, creating lusty sensations against your buttocks and the sensitive areas around your anus and perineum. To make sure you enjoy this position as much as he does, pull his hand around to your clitoris, and encourage him to stroke you. In this position, the blood will rush to your brain, which will either lead to an incredible orgasm or lightheadedness, so be careful.

Vatsyayana, the author of the *Kama Sutra*, comments that this position—also known as Late Spring Donkey by the Taoists—can also be used to imitate the mating of dogs, cats, goats, and deer, as well as "the forcible mounting of an ass, the jump of a tiger, the pressing of an elephant, the rubbing of a boar, and the mounting of a horse." You may find that by imitating mating animals, your own lovemaking will become more primal, more raw. Let your lustiest instincts take over.

JUNE

Tongue Tips (For Her)

Like an especially cute purse, your tongue is the perfect accessory to the perfect blowjob. As you continuously and smoothly bob your head up and down, wiggle your tongue against the ridge on the underside of his shaft. Try a back-and-forth motion. Dip the tip of your tongue into his slit. Circle his entire member. Or, when you reach the top on an upstroke, twist your head a bit, as though you were nodding, and tease your tongue against the *frenulum* (the sensitive strip of skin on the underside of the ridge betweeen his shaft and the head of his penis). Suck on him as though he were a lollipop. Shaking your head while sucking firmly will also produce interesting sensations for him.

While you're in the neighborhood, take a break from his pole to visit the twins. Run your tongue lightly over his testicles. Slip them one at a time into your mouth and suck gently. His perineum, the area between his scrotum and anus, will also respond to the ministrations of your tongue. (This area is also referred to as the taint, as in "'Taint his balls, and 'taint his bum.") If you feel comfortable with this—say you're both freshly bathed—you can even run your tongue between his cheeks, but for safety reasons, you might want to avoid the opening itself unless you're using a barrier of some sort, like a dental dam or even Saran Wrap.

Remember that stopping and re-starting oral treats will heighten his anticipation and generally result in a stronger orgasm when it finally happens. So don't be afraid to pause and pay attention to other parts of his body while you let him cool down a little. You can always use your hands on him until your mouth is ready to work magic on him once again.

JUNE

Tongue Tips (For Him)

Ladies, here's a day's worth of oral sex tips to share with your man. You can even show him this page if you like. Obviously, you'll want him to pleasure you in whatever way makes you happiest.

Guys: "Porno tongue"—sticking it out as far possible as you barely flick her bean—may be a staple of adult films, but it won't do a thing for her except annoy and frustrate. Instead, get your entire mouth involved. Create some buildup. Start out by kissing her belly and thighs, and then work slowly in toward her clit. Explore her entire vulva, including her wet opening. Run your tongue up each side of her clitoral shaft before you begin teasing the bud itself. Swirl around her clitoris. Nuzzle her with your nose. Try a little suction if she likes that. If she's too sensitive for direct stimulation, alternate between circling the bud with a flattened tongue and then a pointy one. Remember that to some women, intense stimulation can quickly become uncomfortable, and once you've reached that point, it's hard to recover.

Here's a key point: If she seems to like what you're doing, *don't stop.* Don't change your speed or pressure. Just keep doing it. Many women need a steady pace, repetition, and constant pressure to climax. If you stop or change what you're doing now, you may distract her, and all your hard work will be for naught. (It can take her anywhere from three minutes to thirty to climb that mountain again.) If you get tired, you can wrap your tongue over your upper lip and move your head, or alternate with a finger. But try to hang in there, and you'll win her undying appreciation.

JUNE

Why Use a Vibrator? Reason #2: Better Partner Sex!

A vibrator isn't just something to use until your partner's available. Many couples include masturbation and toys in their lovemaking with ecstatic results. Sharing vibrators and other sex toys with your man can add spice and variety to your sexual repertoire. Best of all, it can be fun! Barbara, a forty-year-old project manager, happily recounts what happened when her boyfriend took her on an outing to an adult store: "We shared quite a few giggles looking at all of the various toys each one of us could use. Then we each decided on a toy, and the cashier gave us a twenty percent discount, probably because we were having so much fun in the store! We raced home to play with our new toys. I couldn't wait to see him using his, and he couldn't wait to try mine out on me. The combination of all the laughter and the excitement of something new made for a memorable night, as well as more to look forward to!"

As Barbara's experience shows, there's no need for your man to feel threatened by your toy. On the contrary, the excitement, anticipation, and new sensations can enhance sex for both of you. There are lots of toys designed specifically for his enjoyment, as well as several created for you to use together. So don't just assume that your man will be intimidated or jealous if you bring up the subject of incorporating vibrators into your sex life. It's very likely that he'd get a thrill out of seeing you use it on yourself or feeling the sensations on his own body. The key to success is talking about it beforehand. Know that just like a particularly well-adjusted childhood pal, vibrators *do* play well with others.

JUNE

Boyfriend, Meet Vibrator: Introducing Your Man to Your Toy

While you may be dying to share the pleasures of your vibrator with your man, I'd advise against whipping out your Hitachi Magic Wand in the midst of foreplay. Broach the subject beforehand. You can do this in a very sexy way. Tell him that you want to show him how hot you get when you're pleasuring yourself with your toy, and that you fantasize about him using it on you. Most red-blooded men will be panting with curiosity. Here are some other ways to counter concerns:

+ **He'll worry that he hasn't been satisfying me.** Assure him that he has been pleasing you *a lot*, which is why you want to experience even more pleasure with him!

+ **He'll worry that I don't need him anymore.** You can't joke or cuddle with your vibrator, to say nothing of the fact that it's a terrible kisser! Assure him that your vibrator is an accessory to great sex, not a substitute for his warm-blooded super-studly self.

+ **He'll think I shouldn't need something besides him.** If this is the case, gently point out to him that whether it's a fantasy or a setting or a state of mind, everyone "relies" on something other than his or her partner. After all, if he masturbates, he's not relying on you for his pleasure or release, is he?

Ideally, your man won't care how you get off, as long as you *do* get off. If, of course, he's simply worried that he's not able to "give" you orgasms, here's a perfect opportunity to be more open with him about what you need (be more vocal! let him hold the vibrator!)—as well as to point out that your orgasms aren't solely his responsibility. It takes two to tango, after all.

JUNE

Plan a Date Night

All the fancy sex techniques in the world won't help a bit if you don't make time for your lovemaking. This becomes even more important when children enter the picture. On one hand, you'll find that you'll need to be more spontaneous. Take advantage of opportune moments whenever they present themselves, like a child's naptime, or an unexpected play date. Master the art of the quickie. Engage in masturbation or manual and oral manipulation when you can. Things don't always have to lead to intercourse, particularly when you're exhausted.

On the other hand, you may also have to—gasp!—plan for sex. Don't think of it being less spontaneous. *Do* think about the moment when you get to get down and dirty with your main squeeze, and let erotic anticipation build. Listen to Jane, a forty-five-year-old communications manager with two small children:

"The very best thing we've done to stay connected in a romantic way is to have a date night at least one night a week. Because I know it's coming, I get in the mood much more quickly—in fact, I look forward to it all day. This doesn't prevent us from being spontaneous at other times, but it does guarantee at least one time during the week when we're really taking time for each other. It may sound boring, but sexual spontaneity is one of the first casualties of parenthood, so I highly recommend date night!"

Even long-term partners without children can benefit from setting aside time for each other without television (unless it's to watch an erotic video together), computers, or other distractions. Arrange your date night today!

JUNE

Let Him Explore Your Garden

You shouldn't expect to have an orgasm every single time you get busy with yourself or a partner. In fact, it's more likely that expectations will act as an anti-aphrodisiac. Take the pressure off yourself. The best and most reliable way to come is to tell yourself (and mean it) that it's okay if you don't. You can have some incredible erotic experiences if you don't focus on the end goal but on what happens to you on the path. Listen to Cathy, a trainer in her mid-thirties: "If you find that you're not going to climax, that's okay. Some of the most amazingly intimate moments come when you're being touched just for the sheer pleasure of it, instead of being touched for a purpose."

Cathy describes one such experience she had with her man: "He slid the tip of his finger inside me and smeared my wetness around my labia, and then lubricated my clitoris the same way. Then he performed the most sensuous genital massage I've ever experienced, gently stretching out my outer lips one by one and stroking them with his pinky fingers, and rubbing his thumbs tenderly up and down my inner lips. I didn't come, but I'll never forget the experience. It was the most extraordinary attention my genitals had ever received."

As Cathy's story shows, our most memorable erotic encounters often emerge from the attention we give and receive from our lover, the connections we make, and the intimacy we experience—not from whether we've had an orgasm. Remember to enjoy the journey, and you'll open yourself to ecstasy all year long.

CHAPTER SEVEN

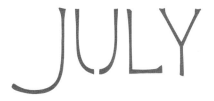

"One swallow does not a summer make."
—*Anonymous proverb*

The sage who came up with this proverb wasn't referring to sex, but that's no reason why we can't use it for our own ends, so to speak, and indulge ourselves this month with a special focus on oral treats. (And we're not talking about Popsicles!) July is a time for vacations, and so this month's tips also encourage you to take a vacation from the thoughts and worries that keep you from fully enjoying your sexual self.

In the late 1800s, people used this month's birth flower, the graceful *larkspur*, to symbolize levity or hilarity. Keep long stems of red, pink, white, and violet larkspurs around your home to remind yourself to lighten up—it's summer!

July's birthstone is the beautiful *ruby*, known as "The King of Gems" by the ancient Hindus. Legend has it that a ruby's red glow comes from an internal fire that can't be put out, making it a perfect symbol of eternal love. Adorn yourself with something ruby-colored this month to remind yourself of Kundalini, the universal creative energy coiled inside you.

JULY

Position of the Week: The Rising Position

This *Kama Sutra* position will definitely get a rise out of him. Lying on your back, raise your legs straight up as your guy kneels in front of you, with his knees close to your derriere, as he enters you. Rest your ankles on either side of his neck. Press your thighs tightly together and push your legs against his shoulders: This squeezes his plunging penis and increases the pressure on it, as well as the sensual friction. If he wants to thrust vigorously, he can hold your legs tightly against his chest for balance.

Fifteen hundred years later, Kalyana Malla, author of the *Ananga Ranga*, described a very similar position called the Level Feet Posture, one of several *uttana-banhda*, or supine positions. The only way this one differs from the Rising Position is that your man lifts your body so that your buttocks are actually resting on his thighs, allowing him to penetrate even more deeply as he ravishes you.

Don't just lie there, though. Even though these positions give him more control, you can still rock your hips, clasp your love muscle and arch your back. The more involved you get, the more pleasure for both of you.

JULY

Keep Your Hands Busy

While your mouth is going to work on your man's love shaft, remember the old saying about idle hands, and keep your paws active. If he is receptive to it, reach up and play with his nipples. Pull, pinch, or rub them gently. Roll them between your fingers. If you're especially good at multi-tasking, tweak his nipples with one hand while you hold or stroke his testicles. And don't forget about the rest of his body, either. Rub his tummy, and massage his inner thighs and the sweet spot where his legs meet his body. Press on his perineum (the area between his scrotum and anus), which will stimulate his prostate. Let him suck on your fingers so he won't feel left out.

Finally, here's a tip my friend Matt says drives his boyfriends wild: During oral sex, slip a well-lubed, manicured finger gently into his bum to massage his anus and prostate. You can also just massage the opening. (For more on this area, and the prostate, see January 30 and April 18.) A straight man of my acquaintance verified Matt's advice: "Not having much anal experience, I was a bit apprehensive, but with lots of lubricant and gentle strokes, my girlfriend took me to a new level of excitement. While going down on me, she slowly inserted her lubed finger into my ass just enough for me to feel her. After adding more lubricant, she timed her finger thrusts with the strokes of her mouth. As I was about to come, she stopped what her mouth was doing and just thrust with her fingers. I had never come so intensely before." Try this sometime, and you'll have a slathering love slave on your hands, perhaps literally.

JULY

More Mouthwork Variations

Another way to give your man a variety of sensations is to alternate your mouth with your vagina. While you're riding his rod, hop off every so often, slide down his body, and play some mouth music. This works best when you're on top, of course. Some men find this particularly exciting, and it will add to your pleasure as well.

Speaking of your pleasure, it's perfectly fine—and very arousing for him—for you to pleasure yourself while you're performing oral sex on him. (Just be sure you can maintain your concentration to some extent.) It's a huge compliment to him: It shows him that you get *so* turned on by sucking on his mansicle that you just can't help but touch yourself. Make sure he gets a good view, which will excite him even more, and let him see you rub your fingers in your wet depths. Imitate what you'd like *him* to be doing inside *you*.

Above all, never forget that men are visual creatures. Keep and maintain eye contact during oral and manual sex so he can see how excited you are. Don't hide behind a curtain of hair, either. Tie back your tresses, or let him hold them back, so he can see what you're doing. Prop up a mirror to give him an even closer look. Be proud of your oral skills!

JULY

Independence Day

Whether you're in a relationship or blissfully sifting through the population, use today to encourage your own sense of independence. It doesn't have to be overtly sexual. Make a date with yourself to do something you love to do—alone. Visit an art museum and spend as much time as you want in your favorite gallery. Get a massage. Go to a spa and sit in the sauna or hot tub for an hour. Steal away to a café with a book or your journal. Treat yourself to an hour of self-loving by your favorite method.

These suggestions draw from a tool that writer Julia Cameron calls an "artist's date" in her book *The Artist's Way.* An artist's date, she says, is "a block of time, perhaps two hours weekly, set aside and committed to nurturing your creative consciousness." Oh, but you're not an artist, you say? Rubbish. Every time you have sex, with yourself or with a partner, you're creating something. Why do you think it's called it "making love?"

But if you're empty inside and disconnected from yourself, you won't have anything to give. By spending time nurturing yourself, you fill your inner well. Later, with your partner or yourself, with your soul nurtured and your batteries recharged, you can make some fireworks together.

JULY

Tongue (His) and Groove (Yours)

Here's one tip to share with your man. Many women find the sensation of being penetrated by their lover's tongue to be pure bliss, as you'll probably agree if you've ever received such a delight. Encourage your man to pretend that his tongue is an especially facile penis. Ask him to tease and probe your wet groove, showing you with his mouth what you'd like him to do with his erection. Urge him to have fun with it by licking around your opening and darting the tip inside. He doesn't have to go deep—remember, most of your nerve endings are in the outer third of your vagina. By breathing gently onto your vulva, he can also warm things up nicely. However, "gently" is the operative word. Blowing air directly into the vagina can, in very rare cases, cause an embolism if there is any damage to the uterine wall. You'd have to blow pretty hard, but still, it's best to be careful.

If you raise your knees toward your chest, you'll really open yourself and give him even better access. And while he has his tongue buried in you, don't be shy about pleasuring your clitoris. He'll be thrilled that you get so carried away. Relax and enjoy the divine sensations, but be sure to let him know you're looking at what he's doing. Your moans of ecstasy will spur him on to higher heights—or in this case, deeper depths.

JULY

Combo Deluxe Platters

Don't be shy about letting him explore your other openings while he's performing mouth music on you. Let him slide a finger or two into your wet vagina while he's teasing your clit! If your man is the kind of guy who can walk and chew gum at the same time, you're set, because it will take some concentration to keep the right pressure going on your love button. Otherwise, you may want to use a dildo or vibrator instead—G-spot stimulation during oral sex can produce some incredible sensations. My friend Annette describes a technique she uses with great results on her girlfriend: "With your palm facing up, place one or two fingers inside her. Curl your fingers like you were telling her to 'come here,' and stroke the area located directly behind the clitoris while you're stimulating it with your mouth. It's guaranteed to work every time!"

If you're both game, encourage him to massage a well-lubed finger around your perineum and the opening of your anus and slowly penetrate you with it. All it might take is him barely entering you to send you over the edge. Communicate with him about what feels best. Do you like slow thrusting, or fast? More than one finger? If you think you'd like a finger or dildo in your vagina as well, let him know. (But be careful that he doesn't mix up his fingers, or put anything that's been in your anus in your vagina, or you could get a nasty bacterial infection.) If the pressure or sensations start feeling too intense, don't just grin and bear it: Let him know to ease up or pull out entirely. It's your combo platter. Have it your way!

JULY

Tanabata: It's in the Stars

On this day, the Japanese celebrate Tanabata, or "star festival," a tradition imported from China in the eighth century. The festival is dedicated to the Cowherd Star (Altair) and Weaver Star (Vega) of the constellations Aquila and Lyra, which are separated by the Milky Way. According to legend, Altair and Vega represent two star-crossed lovers whom the gods allow to meet just once a year, on the seventh day of the seventh month. The Japanese celebrate Tanabata by writing wishes on strips of colored paper and hanging them on the branches of bamboo trees placed in their gardens or the entrances to their homes.

Adapt this tradition to your own sensual purposes. Buy a "lucky bamboo" tree, which these days is fairly easy to come by in most nurseries or Asian markets. If you can't find a bamboo tree, any leafy plant will do. You could even use a bouquet of flowers.

With your lover, jot down up to ten sensual wishes, and hang them from your tree or bouquet using Christmas ornament hooks or colored string. If you like Japanese food, prepare your favorite dish and enjoy it together, expending as much care in the preparation and serving of the meal as you would find in the finest Tokyo restaurant. If you're single, this is a night to pamper yourself.

Then, take turns picking one of the other person's wishes. Do your best, within reason, to make it come true (single folk can do the same for themselves), imagining that you're Altair and Vega and this is the one night of the year that you have together. Memorize your lover's face, his skin, his body, as though 364 days will pass before you see him again.

JULY

Position of the Week: The Pair of Tongs

The *Kama Sutra* notes that when a woman "gets on the top of the man, she then shows all her love and desire." In a position called The Pair of Tongs, you kneel astride your supine lover and draw him into you using your finely toned love muscles. Then, squeeze him repeatedly with your internal "tongs." You can move gently on top of him or simply sit and let both of you reap the benefit of your Kegel exercises.

In fact, now would be a great time to show him the many variations of Kegels you've mastered. Squeeze for three seconds, relax, and repeat. It helps to do this in time with your breathing: Inhale as you contract, hold your breath as you squeeze, then exhale on release. (Ideally, you're doing your Kegels at least ten times at three different times every day.) Or "flutter" your muscles with quickie clenches. If you're a Kegel connoisseur, you can contract your PC muscles starting at the entrance of your vagina and then move to the top, as though there was an elevator inside. Do this several times, and he'll feel like you're milking his love muscle. It's doubtful that you'll hear any complaints.

As the poet Kalyana Malla said much later in the *Ananga Ranga*:

"And she will be pleased to hear that the art once learned, is never lost. Her husband will then value her above all women, nor would he exchange her for the most beautiful Rani (queen) in the three worlds. So lovely and pleasant to man is she who constricts."

JULY

Try the Kivin Method

Unfamiliar with the Kivin method? It's an oral sex technique that seems tailor-made for do-it-yourself men who like to get immediate feedback, and for women who like earth-shattering orgasms. (Is there any woman who doesn't, at least once in a while?) Here's how you do it: First, lie on your back and have your guy lie perpendicular to you. Once you've given him the basic instructions that follow, you get to lie back and enjoy.

Have him put a finger on either side of your clitoral hood and lick back and forth across it (rather than up and down). This avoids possibly too-intense direct stimulation of the clitoris. While he's licking, he presses his middle finger (pad only, no fingernail) on your perineum, the spot midway between your vagina and anus. He'll feel you give involuntary contractions here if he's licking you in the right spot. Help him out by moaning.

Ask him to keep a steady stroke with his tongue and his finger in one place, because if he changes speed or moves his finger, he may distract you. Most importantly, make sure he knows it's okay (assuming it is) to continue past your initial orgasm, because that's often when you'll have the most intense response.

If you want even more intense stimulation—you wild thang, you!—bend your knees up to your chest while he keeps them out of the way with one arm. From here, you'll be wide open to even more pleasure.

JULY

Self-Loving Reason #7: Sweet Dreams!

It's two a.m., and you're wide awake. Worries about work, finances, or the state of your relationship are running around your brain like a hyperactive hamster on a wheel, and the more you think about how you need to fall asleep, the harder it is. You don't want to take medication, because you don't want to feel like a zombie tomorrow. However, there's a natural cure for insomnia that will leave you refreshed, and not stupefied, the next morning—masturbation.

Self-pleasuring to achieve an orgasm is a great way to reduce both physical and emotional tension (see May 2 and June 13 for more on this). Arousal and orgasms activate the painkilling center of your midbrain, which releases waves of hormones (like endorphins) that relax your muscles, reduce anxiety, and calm you down. So next time your racing brain keeps you awake, get busy down below. By the way, the National Center on Sleep Disorders Research encourages insomnia sufferers to associate the bed and bedtime with sleep—which means not using the bed for any activity other than sleep and sex—so if you masturbate to help yourself fall asleep, you're simply following doctor's orders!

Of course, chronic insomnia can be a symptom of an underlying medical condition, like depression or heart disease. If your sleeplessness lasts for weeks or months, please see your doctor, because whether your insomnia is due to a temporary reaction to a stressful situation or an ongoing problem, you should work on treating the root cause. But as a nice quick fix, masturbating tonight can give you a much happier tomorrow.

JULY

Go for a Swim

When the temperature heats up outside, there's nothing more refreshing than a nice dip in the pool, and with a little creativity, you can make your swim downright blissful. In a swimming pool, position yourself over the heating jets. (You can do the same in a jacuzzi or hot tub.) Many women describe the sensation as being similar to a good licking. Be sure you either have privacy or the ability to keep a straight face. And, as always, don't aim the stream directly into your vagina, or you could suffer a fatal air embolism. It's rare, but it happens.

You and your man can have fun splashing around, too. Stand face-to-face in the shallow end, or brace yourself against the edge of the pool. Caress and stroke him until he's ready—if the water's cold, you may need to be a little more diligent with your hand work—and then float into whatever position strikes your fancy. If you're not able to skinny-dip, wear a bikini so you can pull the bottom aside. You can also recreate the rolling-in-the-surf scene in the movie *From Here to Eternity*. If a pool is unavailable, rent a private hot tub room at your fitness club or spa. If you don't want to frolic in the tub, most of these rooms have cots or cushions for you to "rest" on (nudge nudge, wink wink) after a nice long soak.

JULY

Don't Forget to Breathe

Pranayama refers to the formal yogic practice of controlling the breath (*prana* refers to the life force, also known as *chi*). Pranayama is thought by many yogis to be more important than the poses themselves because it acts as a bridge from the *asanas*, or yoga postures, to deeper states of meditation and, ultimately, enlightenment. Practiced diligently, pranayama helps calm, rejuvenate, and revitalize the mind. Controlling the breath can also enhance your lovemaking.

During sex, your breathing naturally speeds up. Breathing consciously and deeply can stimulate you all over and give you stronger, more intense orgasms. Kate, a teacher, describes how breathing helped her focus her mind during sex: "My lover was going down on me, and I decided to put everything out of my mind to focus only on him and what he was doing. As I did this, I watched my breath, just as I do in yoga, concentrating on the inhalation and the exhalation, and the incredible sensations I was feeling. I ended up having the most outrageous full-body orgasm. My entire body was shaking."

If you tend to hold your breath, experiment with inhaling slow deep breaths at any point on the path to achieving orgasms, or try exhaling through your mouth. Practice first by yourself during your next self-pleasuring session so that you get used to the physical sensations. Then, as Kate did, try watching your breath while you're with your partner. When he sees you shuddering with ecstasy, he'll want a tutorial.

JULY

The Grande Finale (His)

So, you've been performing some of these amazing oral sex techniques on your guy, and you get the feeling that he's nearing the finish line. What next? Men often complain that women don't go hard and fast enough at the end, so don't slow down, and don't change what you're doing. Instead, increase your pressure or suction until you've found a speed that works for both of you.

How do you know that he's about to cross the finish line? Ideally, he'll let you know. In addition, his breathing will get heavy, his penis will swell up, his testicles will ascend, and his body will stiffen. When he gets to the point of no return, move your head out of the way and switch quickly to hand work, or simply finish him off with your mouth. After he's done, *stop*. Few men like to be stimulated after they climax (it can actually hurt).

To swallow or not to swallow? Oral sex does *not* count as a safe sex activity. Bodily fluids can transmit HIV and other sexually transmitted diseases, so use a condom. However, if you're in a long-term relationship and sure of each other's health, swallowing his semen can be incredibly erotic and intimate. If you don't care to go this route, you do have options. Slide your mouth off gently after he's done and *discreetly* empty his juices into a washcloth, tissue, or other handy receptacle. You don't want to make him feel self-conscious. After all, you've just taken him to paradise!

JULY

The Grand Finale (Hers)

If you're the happy receiver of your guy's mouth music, be sure you communicate to him what you want him to do when you explode into climax. With many women, the clitoris becomes incredibly sensitive at the moment of an orgasm. If you want him to stop stimulating you, tell him. Let him know whether he should keep putting pressure on you, hold you gently in his mouth, or let go altogether. Of course, you might want to give him these pointers when you're not in the throes of passion.

Hopefully, you're blessed with a patient lover who knows that three minutes of licking isn't going to do it. It is possible, however, that you might psych yourself out, so try to put worries and distractions out of your mind. Instead focus on the sensations, and surrender to them. If you're used to being in control, let yourself go. It's okay to writhe about. You don't look stupid—you look sexy. If you're worried that he's going to get tired, stop it. You can always make sure he has lots of pillows to prop up your hips or his chest. Encourage him to try things like wagging his head—this keeps his tongue on you—or using his finger every once in a while.

If, despite all his oral attention, you know you're not going to come, don't feel bad. Some days it just isn't gonna happen. If you pressure yourself, you'll only make it harder for the next time. Let him know how much you enjoyed yourself, give him a "A" for effort, and move on to the next course.

JULY

Position of the Week: The Ninth Posture

The Ninth Posture of *The Perfumed Garden* is one of those two-for-the-price-of-one rear entry positions. In this position, you kneel on the floor while leaning forward onto your bed or couch—or stand, leaning over a table or other horizontal surface—as your lover enters you from behind. If you enjoy G-spot stimulation, this is your position, because it allows the deepest level of penetration at exactly the right angle. You can change the depth of penetration and the G-spot intensity by raising yourself up on your hands.

This position features prominently in many people's fantasies of going at it over the dining room table, an office desk, or other horizontal surface, and it's not hard to see why. It lends itself perfectly to passionate, devil-may-care quickies: You can do it with your clothes off, or just pushed to one side. Your man will love the stimulation to the head of his penis and the sensation of his thighs (and possibly his scrotum) slapping against your delicious backside. He can also reach around and massage your clitoris—or you can do it yourself if he's holding onto your hips for dear life. You can even get creative and lay your favorite vibrator on the bed against your sweet spot, with your body weight holding it in place.

JULY

Why Use a Vibrator? Reason #3: The Variety!

Vibrators come in a truly amazing assortment of sizes, shapes, and even colors. Want a vibrator that doubles as an all-over massager? Try the Hitachi Magic Wand. Got thin walls and need something quiet? Try a coil vibrator. Want fun in the shower or tub? Look for a waterproof vibe. Want to give him the reins? Get one with a remote control.

Vibrators also offer several kinds of stimulation, with rotating shafts and clitoral vibes, like the famous Rabbit Pearl, which features tumbling plastic pearls in its rotating midsection and two rabbit ears that flicker against your clitoris. There are vibrators to stimulate your G-spot, and others that titillate your tush. There are even vibes that fit over your finger, turning any digit into an instrument of pleasure. Some tiny "bullet" vibes are small enough to fit in the palm of your hand, and they come with a plethora of fun attachments. Speaking of fun, you can even find vibrators to appeal to your sense of humor. The Hot Lips Vibe looks like a tube of lipstick; another vibe looks like a rubber duckie; there's even one with Hello Kitty on the top.

The point is that there's no reason to feel that you're going to be forced to buy something that's shaped or looks like a penis. If that's what you want, great, but can you imagine going to a restaurant and only finding steak on the menu? Take time to explore the wide world of vibrators to find the exact style—or styles—that's right for you.

JULY

This Mortal Coil

Coil-operated vibrators resemble small hair dryers or handheld electric mixers. Usually about six or seven inches long, they feature a small protruding nub on which you can attach a variety of fun attachments. The vibrations come from an electromagnetic coil inside that also accounts for the vibrator's relative heaviness. Coil vibrators vary slightly between manufacturers—the best-known is Wahl—and usually allow only two choices of speeds: low and high (a.k.a "Oh my!" and *Oh my God!*).

Plug in a coil vibrator if noise is an issue either because you have thin walls, or you just don't want to listen to the sound of heavy machinery when you're pleasuring yourself. Using one is pretty straightforward: Just place the desired attachment on the metal nub and turn it on. You should be barely able to hear it. Just as with a wand vibrator, you might want to work up to genital stimulation. Start out using it for its stated purpose—as a body massager—as you warm up your genitals with the other hand. When you're relaxed and aroused, apply the vibrating tip to your clitoris and vulva, and revel in the intense, focused sensations.

JULY

Extreme Makeover—for Your Vibrator

Do you love "before and after" shows? Then you'll adore the options your coil-operated vibrator gives you, because most come with several different attachments. For example, the popular Wahl coil comes with seven different attachments. The "spot massager," which sports a small rounded tip, is perfect for teasing your clitoris (dip it into the wetness of your vaginal opening, too). Try the suction cup attachment on your little jewel or your nipples; hold the cup over your finger to turn it into a vibrating toy. And the "scalp stimulator" attachment can be used on many more places than just your head.

Stores like Good Vibrations sell an entire coil attachment kit like the Clitickler, which does exactly what the name implies. This vibe's curved attachment is great for titillating your G-spot, and the straight attachment works well if you're using the vibrator in different positions. Do *not* use these for anal play: if they pop off, they could slip into your rectum. However, there is one attachment shaped like a twig— a branch designed for clitoral stimulation branches off the main shaft—that could be used anally, because the branch will keep it from getting lost in your bum.

Also keep in mind that your wand vibrator doesn't need to be left out of this makeover madness. Both vinyl and silicone attachments are available for the Hitachi Magic Wand. The G-spotter offers a slim, curved probe that works for both goddess-spot massage and prostate stimulation; while the "wonder wand" lets you send the wand's vibration deep inside. Dress up your vibrator today—you both deserve it!

JULY

Awakening the Fourth Chakra

The fourth, or heart, chakra nourishes our feelings of love, affection, and compassion. This chakra becomes blocked by unhealed emotional wounds as well as emotions such as heartbreak, grief, and longing. But if you can open and re-awaken this chakra, love will flow out of you naturally like a mountain spring. To help you do that, here's a version of a technique outlined by my co-author David Ramsdale in our book *Red Hot Tantra.* It harnesses the explosive sexual energy in your second, or sex, chakra, and unifies it with your heart center in order to open both. Try it by yourself first, then with a partner.

First, pleasure yourself until you're just on the edge of having an orgasm. Get close, but don't let go. Do this at least three times, imagining a tube of energy between your genitals and your heart. Mentally touch your chest between your nipples. If you like, touch yourself physically in this spot with your free hand.

Then, when you're ready to climax, press the palm of your hand to your chest and rub. Imagine light shooting up the tube from your sexual energy center to your heart. You may want to repeat the word "Love!" or "Yam!" (the mantra for the heart center) or another word that works for you. Roll your head back and *let yourself go.* Surrendering your sense of control is critical if you want to experience the full bliss not only of lovemaking, but of connecting with another human being as well. Abandon yourself to the sensations coursing through your veins—and the love flowing through and out of your heart.

JULY

Ring Around the Rosy

The ways to please a man's love wand with your hands are virtually endless. Remember the ring you made around his penis with your thumb and index finger to enhance oral sex on June 20? The same move can be used during manual labor.

Keep a tight grip, especially as you pop over his ridge. Or make two rings—put them in the middle of his penis—and stroke outwards, in opposite directions. A similar method is to slide the "ring" upwards from the base toward the tip. Just as it reaches the top, repeat the motion with the other hand so that you're starting at the base just as the other hand reaches the tip. This can produce a very powerful and explosive orgasm, so be prepared.

Another writer gave me a tip adapted from a technique many men use on themselves: "With one hand, grasp the base of his penis firmly using an O-shaped grip. With your other hand, spiral toward the top, giving extra attention to the head as your palm and fingers pass over it. When he's about to experience an orgasm, place both hands just below the tip and use strong circular motions to 'pop his cork.'" If you're super-coordinated, try spiraling both hands toward the top!

JULY

A Helping Hand... or Two

When you're giving your man a helping hand, why not give him two? While sitting in front of him, wrap your fingers around his penis with your fingers laced together. Twist this way and that, with slight up-and-down squeezing motions, or put your hands together with your palms and fingertips touching. Slide the base of your palms down over his shaft. Every so often, let his penis poke out between your fingers, keeping those nearest you pressed against the ridge on the underside of his shaft. Let him slip up between your thumbs and index fingers, and then press on the ridge with your thumbs in circular motions. Using both hands can be helpful if he's not quite hard yet.

You can also practice the following technique, which is similar to one of the "ring" techniques we discussed yesterday. Grasp his entire shaft with your hand and squeeze gently upwards. As you reach the tip, repeat the same motion with the other hand. Keep going, as though you were descending a fire pole. To vary this, grasp his penis with both hands and twist slowly up and down as you move your wrists in opposite directions. You can use this same motion with your index finger and thumb. Just don't "wring" him too hard, and whatever you do, don't forget the lube!

JULY

Position of the Week: Ananga Ranga Side-by-Side Positions

When you've been having lots of high-impact, high-energy sex, side-by-side positions can offer you a nice break without making you stop completely. Since neither partner is on top, it's also probably a good bet for those who want to dispense with power issues and get all warm and fuzzy once in a while.

The *Ananga Ranga* lists three side-by-side positions, which are referred to as *tiryak-bandha*, or transverse, positions. With the Transverse Lute, you both stretch your legs out straight: Lift one leg so that he can enter you, then guide his top leg onto your top thigh (bend your knee slightly). Or you can stretch your legs out straight in the Cupped Position. You'll feel his thrusts against the inside of your labia, which are pressed against his legs. If he scoots up a little toward your head, the base of his penis may even pleasure your clitoris.

The *Ananga Ranga* is quiet on the subject, but the *Kama Sutra* says that the man should lie on his left side with the woman on her right. If your man's right-handed and wants to stimulate your love button, this probably makes sense, but if he's left-handed, by all means switch sides. Of course, any and all free hands should be busy exploring each other's face, arms, torso, and the rest of the body. Wouldn't it be nice to fall asleep so intertwined?

JULY

I Am Leo, Hear Me Roar

If your birthday falls between July 23 and August 22, your sign is Leo, represented by a lion. Generous and warmhearted by nature, Leos love being the center of attention. They also love the high life—and believe they deserve the very best. If you're just starting a relationship with a Leo, make sure your finances are in order and that you have lots of discretionary income. Now is not the time to show your frugal side. Think quality—and, if you can afford it, quantity.

Seduce your Leo by appealing to his sense of theatricality. (If you're the Leo, this will get your motor running, too.) Make reservations at a hot new restaurant where you can see and be seen. Start your foreplay over dinner by whispering things you want to do to him as you stroke his thigh. List one item at a time, and end each item with a kiss on the ear and neck. Make this even sexier by literally purring in his ear. As my friend Mick, a writer in his forties, advises, "Learn to purr like Catwoman. For some reason, this just works. Maybe it's from growing up watching *Batman.* Maybe it's from seeing Michelle Pfeiffer in that Catwoman outfit. I don't know. But it works." After dinner, suggest a little walk, and every time you reach a corner, lean over to kiss him and tell him how you can't wait to get him home. Each time, end with a purr.

Don't overdo it, of course. A breathy whisper is preferable if you can't quite get the purr right. Just let your Leo know, in your huskiest voice, that when he gets you home he's going to have a wildcat on his hands.

JULY

Uddiyana Bandha, the Abdominal Lock

For the next two days, we're going to build on the July 12 tip by talking about two different types of *pranayama*, or breathing techniques. Many people dismiss these breathing exercises, but they're missing out.

Today's technique, the *Uddiyana Bandha* or abdominal lock, can soothe and revitalize your internal organs and digestive system, and replace a sluggish mind with an alert, energized one. It can also raise your sexual energy by strengthening the nerves and muscles in your lower belly, thereby increasing your orgasmic potential. Start by sitting quietly in a cross-legged position with your palms on your knees. (You should also have an empty stomach.) Let your breath slow down. Breathe in deeply, letting your belly expand; hold, and then exhale completely until no air remains in your lungs.

When you're ready, inhale again, and then exhale forcefully through your nose and pull your belly in and up under your ribcage (your upper abdomen will "hollow out"). Tighten your PC and anal muscles. Hold your breath in this "locked" position for as long as possible before inhaling slowly through your nose and softening your belly. Take a few deep, slow breaths and let your breathing go back to normal before you try another round. Begin your practice with three rounds, then work up to ten.

You may get a slight head rush from practicing Uddiyana Bandha. If it lasts for more than a few minutes, you might be doing too many rounds of the breath. Scale back for a bit.

NOTE: Please don't try this exercise if you're pregnant or have high blood pressure, heart disease, or glaucoma. Also *do not* practice any pranayama exercise if you've been drinking alcohol or taking drugs.

JULY

Fire Breath

Kapalabhati pranayama, also known as the "Breath of Fire" in Kundalini yoga, will help you clear your mind, and both purify and energize your body before lovemaking. A side effect is that it's also purported to encourage stronger and better orgasms! Please start slow when you're doing these exercises, which are considered advanced techniques in some yogic traditions.

Similar to Uddiyana, the Fire Breath consists of several rounds of rapid diaphragmatic breathing featuring an active, forced exhalation with a passive inhalation. Sit in a comfortable seated position. As you inhale through your nose, let your belly swell. Then exhale forcefully through your nose several times—five or ten the first time—pulling your belly up as though you were pressing it into your spine and up into your rib cage. It's like using your belly to try to blow a candle out through your nose. In fact, put your hand on your belly to make sure it's pumping.

After your last quick exhalation, hold the out-breath for as long as is comfortable. If you want, you can hold your next inhalation, too. Then let your breathing return to normal. You should have more energy; if you feel lightheaded, stop. If you want to try the Fire Breath during sex, do it during a rest break and then go back to the action. With regular practice, the Fire Breath can help you have orgasms that are, if you'll excuse the pun, truly breathtaking!

NOTE: Please don't try this exercise if you have your period, are pregnant, have high blood pressure, or have had recent abdominal surgery. And again, *do not* try this if you've been taking drugs or drinking alcohol.

JULY

A Vacation from Inhibitions

July is a time when many people look forward to vacations from their everyday lives. Today, give yourself a vacation from the inhibitions that keep you from enjoying your full sexual potential. Number one: Don't be shy about pleasuring yourself during intercourse. Let yourself get carried away! He'll find it incredibly sexy if you're so turned on by the feeling of him inside you that you can't keep from touching yourself. If the end result is mind-blowing ecstasy for both of you, who's going to complain!

Woman-on-top, rear entry, and spooning positions lend themselves quite well to self-pleasuring. In fact, the rear entry and spoon positions might be a good place to start, because you won't be facing him and your hands will be free to play with yourself. He'll love to feel you get progressively more excited. Why not show off your skills when you're on top? Lean back and massage your clitoris as you ride him. Then wet your finger and massage your lust-hardened nipple as he watches in fascination. While you're at it, you can always give his glistening member a few strokes no matter what position you're in.

Don't hog the fun to yourself, though. Have him put his hand over yours so he can feel exactly what you're doing. Ideally, he'll learn a thing or two.

JULY

Give Yourself a Masturbation Makeover

Granted, most of us have a dependable masturbation routine that probably suits us just fine. Why mess with a good thing? Because it will help you have *more* good things—more orgasms, that is. Masturbating with different methods increases your options for pleasure and teaches you more about your sexual response. You'll also have more freedom to decide where, when, and how you want to come. You don't *always* have to be on your back in bed with your favorite vibrator. (Like, what if you just finished this year's *Best American Erotica* and your body is screaming for release, but you're in a 747 at 10,000 feet somewhere over the Atlantic?) Another benefit is that your partner will have a better chance of pleasing you in a variety of ways. Finally, if you don't depend on one method of climaxing, you'll be better prepared as your body changes over the years.

So how do you change your style? Be patient with yourself. Deprive yourself of your favorite methods, and set aside some time to experiment. Do it in front of the mirror—or in front of your partner. Experiment with different breathing patterns or change positions. If you always lie on your back, try flipping over or sitting up. If you're always quiet, make noise. Thrash around. Seduce yourself with warm oil, silk sheets, and candles. Steal your boyfriend's lube or buy your own water-based brand. And try a new fantasy. A sordid new mental adventure may be your ticket to new delights.

JULY

Shower à Deux

When the thermometer rises, it's sometimes hard to think about getting all hot and sticky with your man. So why not cool down together, in a lukewarm or cool shower? Tell him you're going to go cool off and then accidentally "drop" your towel as you head for the shower. If he doesn't get the hint, invite him in. Once the water's flowing over the two of you, have fun. Wash each other's hair. Soap each other up with a fragrant, invigorating shower gel. Using a washcloth or bath mitt, lather his chest and move down his body to soap his penis and family jewels.

If he's not standing at attention yet, rinse him off, kneel, and take him in your mouth. The sight of your slick body kneeling in front of him will be a huge turn-on (and he can do the same for you as well). Once he's hard, rub his penis against your slippery buttocks and vagina. Then turn away from him and bend over slightly so he can enter you from behind. This position will allow you to brace yourself so you don't trip—just be sure you have a bath mat! A fun alternative to intercourse is masturbating each other with the jets of water from the showerhead or shower massager.

Beth, a thirty-two-year-old project manager, comments, "I love taking a long shower in the dark with candles. The running water adds intimacy and closeness!"

JULY

Position of the Week: The Fitter-In

Here's a nice position from *The Perfumed Garden* that's perfect for a lusty summer picnic. As your man sits on the ground with his legs outstretched, sit down on him, intertwining your right thigh over his left thigh, and your left thigh over his right. Grasp his upper arms as he grasps yours, and pull yourself onto his erection. Now, you both rock gently back and forth—"moving with little concussions," says the author Sheikh Nefzawi—keeping your rhythm by pressing your feet onto the ground. Imagine you're in your own private playground, riding a most delightful swing.

While you're here, you might try one of the "movements of love" described by the *Perfumed Garden*'s author. For example, there's "The Mutual Shock," in which each of you pull back without dislodging his penis entirely, and then push together tightly once again. Or make "The Approach," in which your man thrusts and stops, and then you do the same. Both movements seem well suited to this artistic, rocking position.

JULY

Can You Hum a Few Bars?

You've probably heard blowjobs referred to as "hummers." Well, let's take that literally. While you have him in your mouth, moan or hum lightly. This creates a vibration in your mouth that will feel quite nice on his penis. He can do the same to you, too, while he's sucking your love button. Essentially, humming turns you into a human vibrator. And, if your vibrating moans come about because you're getting into what you're doing, it's even more exciting.

Some Tantric experts have actually suggested humming the Sanskrit word "Om" during oral sex as a way to worship your loved one's lingam or yoni and recognize its divine nature. Usually used during meditation, Om is a mantra, a sacred word repeated to facilitate higher states of consciousness. In Hinduism, Om (also called Aum, because it combines the sound "Ah," "Oh," and "Mm") is the most sacred syllable. It is considered to have accompanied creation; Hindus believe that it is the sound of the universe continuing to vibrate. You might find that humming or chanting Om, whether during sex or as part of a meditation ritual, makes you feel more energetic and connected. Allow the sound to vibrate throughout your entire body.

Some people might feel silly about chanting. Think of it instead as a tool for focusing your mind, and clearing out the chatter so that you can focus on the heightened sense of awareness that comes with sensual lovemaking.

JULY

Treats for Your Taste Buds

Why not finish off the month with tasty treats? Blueberries, peaches, nectarines, plums—summer is the season for fresh fruit. Take the time to indulge your oral fixation in more ways than one, by turning your bodies into living fruit platters. Nibble a blueberry out of his bellybutton. Spoon strawberries and cream into each other's mouths and then trace the cream around your bodies. My friend Anne advises, "Have your partner go to work on you with chilled peach slices—all around, in and out." Imagine what you could do with a frozen banana! Or a popsicle turned into a spur-of-the-moment dildo! Give either a couple of sexy sucks with your mouth, and then rub them between your vaginal lips.

Turn his penis into a big fruitsicle: puree some mango, bananas, or papaya, apply it to his member, and take some time licking it off. Douse him with caramel or whipped cream. Drizzle him with melted (but cooled) chocolate. Then put a spoonful of your favorite ice cream in your mouth, and slide him in your mouth. You'll have a life-sized ice cream sundae, and the sensation of the cold on his hot member will give him a tasty sensation he won't forget. Turn your body into a dessert tray, too. Trace honey, whipped cream, or caramel around your nipples and draw a line down to your clitoris, or tuck berries into your vaginal lips, and invite him in for a snack.

CHAPTER EIGHT

AUGUST

"Shall I compare thee to a summer's day?
Thou art more lovely and more temperate.
Rough winds do shake the darling buds of May,
And summer's lease hath all to short a date."
—*William Shakespeare (1564-1616),* Sonnet 18

This month's tips will describe ways that you can enjoy the end of summer through relaxing sensual rituals *and* super-hot techniques with props like ice cubes! The "hot" theme will continue with more tips on using vibrators to enhance your erotic play, and because Good Vibrations has designated August as National Anal Sex Month, this month will offer a few suggestions for enjoying anal sex play safely.

This month's birth flowers are the *gladiolus* and the *poppy.* The Victorians gave each other gladioli to symbolize love at first sight, and red poppies to represent pleasure. Even if you're in a long-term relationship, you might use a cut stem of gladiolus blossoms to remind yourself to look at your love with new eyes, and a bouquet of poppies as a cue to enjoy pleasures both simple and extravagant.

The *peridot,* a beautiful, transparent lime or olive green stone, is August's birthstone. Called the "evening emerald" by the Romans, peridots were said to help dreams become reality. Wear a pretty peridot as a symbol this month, and you'll make your dreams come true.

AUGUST

Road Trip!

Summer is the season for vacations long and short, so hop in your car for a little road trip! Head for an empty freeway or secluded country road where your privacy's assured—the last thing you want is a police officer tapping on your window just as things get hot and heavy.

If you want to think of your car as your own mobile bedroom, remember one caveat: Foreplay on the road (if at all), orgasms on the roadside. When your man is driving, rev his engines by rubbing or tapping him through his pants. Stroke yourself but don't let him look. Wait until you've stopped before working his member out of his pants—or guiding his hand to your nether regions—or before giving yourself a full-blown orgasm. Be sure that the driver's attention is on the road *at all times* while the vehicle is moving.

Once you've stopped the car someplace safe where you're not going to be interrupted, it's time to get busy. Lean over and take him in your mouth. Put him in the passenger seat and mount him with your knees on either side of his hips or over the back of the seat if it's tilted back. Or face away from him. Crawl into the back seat together and have at it. If you truly are in a secluded spot, get out, hop up onto the trunk of the car, lean back, and have him drive his piston into you. Just make sure the engine's cooled down, because *you'll* be getting hot.

AUGUST

"I am not in this world to live up to other people's expectations,
nor do I feel that the world must live up to mine."
—Frederick "Fritz" Perls, German-born psychologist
and founder of Gestalt therapy

A Vacation from Expectations

Expectations are traps. They keep you on a narrow, proscribed path and cheat you out of the joys of the unexpected. Expectations are different from hope. Expectation says, "This sex had better be good, or I'm going to be pissed off." Hope says, "Gee, I hope that my lover and I have a good time in bed. I'm sure we will, no matter what happens." Hope embraces possibility, leaving you open and free.

What expectations do you have about sex? The media showers us with messages that may or may not be appropriate for you. Do you expect yourself to always be in the mood? Do you expect sex to happen at certain times or in certain ways? Do you expect yourself to always be able to "give" your lover an orgasm—or vice versa? Today, take a vacation from those expectations. Let yourself be open to whatever happens. Try to eliminate the word "should" from your vocabulary. With the exception of discussions about safe sex, the tips in this book are just that—tips. If one works for you and gives you something fun to try, great. If not, skip it and go to another day.

What expectations do you have about your orgasms? Try letting go of preconceived notions and view an orgasm, of any type, as a *possible* result of sexual activity, but not the goal. If you're not focusing on the destination, you'll be much freer to enjoy the variety of subtle pleasures along the way.

AUGUST

Making Condoms Sexy

If you haven't been living in a cave for the past twenty-odd years, you know that condoms are a non-negotiable part of sex, unless you're in an HIV-negative, monogamous relationship and use a reliable form of birth control.

So, no more whining about condoms being unsexy and uncomfortable. Thanks to innovations in technology, they *can* be comfortable (see September 13), and it's your *attitude* that can make them sexy. Look at it in a glass-more-than-half-full kind of way: a condom means that sex is imminent. You're about to get *laid!* Make it part of the action, just like you'd dim the lights or get into a more comfortable position before you start knocking boots for real. Ask him if you can help him put it on, teasing him as you go—or let him make putting it on an erotic show for you.

For example, you could thrill him by putting it on with your mouth. Make an "O" with your lips, and put a slightly unrolled condom between your lips, in front of your teeth. (Be sure the condom's facing the right way; also, you might want to use an unlubricated one.) Holding his erection with one hand, place your mouth at the top. Tighten your lips and slowly push down along the shaft. Now that he's properly dressed, get ready to play!

AUGUST

Position of the Week: Coital Alignment Technique

Despite what today's movies, romance novels, and porn films might indicate, fewer than thirty percent of women can climax from intercourse alone. The vast majority require some sort of stimulation to the clitoris. However, the clitoris and the vaginal opening are just far enough apart that thrusting into a woman's vagina with a penis or dildo isn't going to do the trick. The Coital Alignment Technique (CAT) is a scientific-sounding name for a method designed to remedy this situation.

Basically, the CAT is missionary sex with your man thrusting at just the right angle for his penis to stimulate your love button. First, he enters you slightly (just the head of his penis should be in), and moves up your body so that his shaft makes contact with your mons. His legs should be straight, with yours outstretched and wrapped around his thighs, and with your ankles on his calves. He then slips his hands under your armpit until he's cupping your shoulders.

Now, instead of him thrusting, you begin slowly rocking your hips. Tilt your pelvis away from him so that his penis almost slides out and the base presses against your clit. Then he rocks his pelvis to enter you fully as you tilt back up, squeezing your thighs and PC muscles. Repeat. Each time he pulls out, he slides forward, toward the head of the bed. If this sounds complicated, just remember that the idea is to keep the base of his penis in constant pressure with your clitoris. It might take some practice to get the rhythm right, but that could be part of the fun!

AUGUST

Stop! Do Not Enter!

Sometimes, we forget that it *is* possible to have sex without intercourse. Don't be so focused on penetration—yes, that goes for both ladies and gents—that you forget about the other delights along the way. There can be very real reasons to try alternatives to intercourse: You're just not ready; you forgot the condoms; you have tremendous self-control and believe that delaying gratification is good for the soul.

For example, take "dry humping." What could be more of a turn-on than rubbing your bodies together and feeling his erection through your clothes or against your skin? Rub your clitoris against any part of his body: thigh, hip, pubic bone, or knee. The Coital Alignment Technique described yesterday can be adapted quite successfully to intercourse without penetration. Your sweetie lies on top of you, bracing himself on his elbows, his legs between yours. He's just high enough so that his penis rubs against your clitoris. Then, with both of you bracing your feet against the end of the bed, you rub your bellies back and forth until ecstasy ensues. Your hands should feel free to roam about his body during the action.

NOTE: Unless your man is wearing a condom, this is probably not a safe-sex move because it is possible that some of his pre-ejaculate, or actual ejaculate, could come in contact with your bodily fluids. Be safe.

AUGUST

Invest in Your Mutual Fun

Self-pleasuring with your partner, also known as mutual masturbation, has several things going for it. For one, it's ideal safe sex. For another, it's a great alternative to intercourse if you're in a tight spot—a compact car, seats 22A and 22B of an airplane, a pup tent—or one (or both) of you just aren't in the mood to go all the way. You get to play voyeur and exhibitionist at the same time, and you get to stimulate yourself exactly the way you like. As a variation to your usual routine, mutual masturbation can be lots of fun.

One of the best things about tossing off together is the sheer educational value. You get to show your man exactly what sort of movement, pressure and speed you like, and he gets to do the same. And because you have to let your guard down to let your lover see you pleasuring yourself, mutual masturbation requires trust and caring. It can draw you closer, and make you more comfortable with each other.

So have fun with your simultaneous self-loving session. Sit at opposite ends of the bed and watch each other. Sit in front of a mirror. Time your orgasms so you come together, or take turns. Try it in different positions. Use it as foreplay or the main event. Make out while doing it. Get out your favorite toys. And take mental notes—you might learn a thing or two.

AUGUST

Self-Loving Reason #8: It Puts You in Charge!

The beauty of masturbation is that you control where, when, and how you have your orgasms, or whether you have one at all. Knowing what it takes to make yourself climax makes it easier to show your man exactly what to do in order to bring you to ecstasy.

Self-pleasuring also reminds us that we can be fully sexual beings with or without a partner. You don't have to depend on a man for your pleasure. I'm not knocking partner sex—far from it. Loving relationships are tremendously fulfilling and joyous, but many women feel as though they're not complete unless they're in a relationship, so they spend all their time looking for one. We've all been there. Ironically, when you stop looking for a relationship and start enjoying your independence, partners pop out of the woodwork.

What does this have to do with masturbation? Well, masturbation is a microcosm of your independence. When you pleasure yourself, you're free to imagine yourself with a lover who satisfies your every whim, or simply enjoy your body and its marvelous capacity for sensation. There's no need to look outside yourself—the potential for ecstasy lies within, and you hold the key.

AUGUST

A Taste of Brazil

Summer means bathing suits, and bathing suits, for most women, mean bikini waxing. With a Brazilian bikini wax, the hair is removed from your entire pubic region, including the mons, outer labia, and down into the crease between your buttocks. Some women leave a little patch in the front; others remove everything.

What should you expect when you go for a Brazilian wax? You might be given a paper thong, but chances are that you'll be nude below the waist. Don't worry: Your aesthetician has seen it all. Expect to contort your lower body into a variety of positions so that she can reach every nook and cranny. Afterwards, she may tweeze any remaining stray hairs. The pain? I'm not going to kid you: For a few seconds, it stings like hell, but if you pull the skin to hold your labia tight, it will hurt much less. And it will be over in less than fifteen minutes. To find an aesthetician, ask around. Prices range from $35 to $80 and up.

A Brazilian bikini wax is a sexy surprise for your man. If the thought of hot wax down there makes you wince, turn it into an erotic event and ask him to shave you down there. (Make sure he takes lots of time slathering you with baby oil afterwards.) Once you're newly smooth, guide his hand between your legs and watch his eyes widen. Being smooth will also produce some interesting new sensations for you during oral sex and lovemaking. If you don't like it, you can always grow it back.

AUGUST

Getting Started with Backdoor Play

Thanks to the high concentration of nerve endings in this part of your body, anal play can be erotic, fun, and highly satisfying. Many men find that stimulation of their prostate gland results in incredible orgasms, while women enjoy different yet equally intense sensations. Dawn, a twenty-five-year-old editorial assistant, says, "I think it's very likely that there's a G-spot there, because I have the most explosive orgasms with anal sex." Since it requires relaxing an area that can hold considerable tension, some even find anal penetration to be a soothing, almost meditative experience.

The most common inhibition about anal activity is squeamishness about hygiene. As we discussed back in January, the rectum is a passageway, not a storage area, so if you've gone to the bathroom recently (yet another reason for a high-fiber diet), there shouldn't be more than traces of feces. Take a shower or bath together, using a soapy finger to gently clean the area. If you must use an enema, replace the chemical solution with lukewarm water, or simply try a few squirts with an ear syringe.

The second fear people have is disease. Remember, viruses—not practices—cause disease, and it's unprotected sex of any kind that makes virus transmission more likely. That's why condom use is *de rigueur* for anal play, unless you and your partner have both tested negative for HIV and STDs. Besides, using a condom can banish any lingering worries about cleanliness. Wash *everything* that goes spelunking in your bum both before and after, and *never* put anything that's been in your bottom anywhere else without cleaning it first. Following these simple precautions will let you explore your backdoor with confidence and pleasure!

AUGUST

It's All About You

Every once in a while, it's nice to give each other a vacation from being selfless in the sack. If you don't have to think about the other person's pleasure, you might find it easier to relax and surrender to your body's responses. Turn it into a game: On alternate nights, focus completely on the other person. When it's your man's turn, make sure he doesn't have to lift a finger unless it's to tell you what he likes. Tie him to the bed, if you must, to prove that it's all about him. The next night, it's your turn.

Since most people get turned on by seeing their lover aroused—and by knowing that they're the one who did it—the giver gets a hot little ego boost, and the recipient gets to lie back without worrying about reciprocating, which frees him or her to enjoy the sensations. Amelia, a thirty-four-year-old financial planner, says this allows her to clear her mind of the day's "stuff" and "tune into my body, feelings, breathing, and the feeling of skin touching skin, as well as my partner's breathing, movements, warmth, and the bristle of his hairy legs and chest." When her lover whispers her name in her ear just before reaching an orgasm, it sends her right over the edge.

On your night, notice whether it's hard for you to receive all of the attention. Many women are conditioned to be pleasers; for one evening, let yourself get over it. Let your inner diva emerge. Imagine how studly your guy will feel knowing he's the one who can give you intense pleasure. Relax, and let him.

AUGUST

Position(s) of the Week: Fixing of a Nail and Other Acrobatic Positions

Many of the positions described in the *Kama Sutra* seemed designed to be approached with playfulness. How else to explain some of the more acrobatic missionary poses Vatsyayana describes? Take, for example, the Fixing of a Nail. As your man enters you from a kneeling position, raise one of your legs, but instead of resting it on his shoulder, as in the Splitting of a Bamboo, touch your heel gently against his forehead. As he thrusts, the movements of your raised leg will change the sensations between penis and vagina. It's unclear if the name of the pose refers to the line of your leg, or the act itself, but Vatsyayana definitely had a poetic appreciation for the shapes that lovers' bodies make together, even if he did advise that this position is "learnt by practice only."

Then there's the Crab's Position, where you bend your knees and draw in your legs like a crab pulling in its claws. The motion will constrict your vagina around his member like a silken vise.

Students of yoga—or other particularly flexible women—can experiment with the Lotus-Like Position, although it may leave you feeling somewhat like a pretzel. Lying on your back, raise your legs and cross them into the Lotus pose, ankles resting on the tops of your thighs, as he enters you. Don't worry if you can't achieve this position or keep it for very long. Just keep your sense of humor. Look at these positions as play. Perhaps Vatsyayana intended these positions to be reminders that sex is fun!

AUGUST

Why Use a Vibrator? Reason #4: It's Natural!

Occasionally, people claim that the use of vibrators is unnatural, as though we shouldn't engage in sex using anything man-made. If you took this argument to its logical conclusion, we wouldn't eat with utensils, go out wearing clothes, or travel from place to place in cars. Sure, vibrators aren't strictly necessary for sex. Neither is kissing, but they both make it a lot more pleasurable.

People also claim that using a vibrator is "artificial." How can anything that lets us explore and enjoy our bodies' natural sexual impulses and tactile sensations be artificial? Does this mean that massage oil, satin sheets, candlelight, and soft music are artificial, too? Yes, but we don't feel badly about using them. One of the greatest joys of being human is enjoying tactile stimulation, and there's nothing unnatural about an instrument that helps you become more in tune with your body's delicious sexual responses. Many women need the consistent pressure and stimulation of a vibrator to climax, so what would *really* be unnatural is depriving yourself of the God-given ecstasy of an orgasm.

Some people are threatened by vibrators, but those of us who use them know that our toy will never replace another flesh-and-blood human being. While they'll never break your heart (unless the batteries suddenly die), vibrators can't laugh with you, they can't cry with you, and they're terrible at spooning into your naked skin on a warm summer night. But vibrators can help you enjoy your sexuality during those times when you don't have a partner in your life, and there's nothing unnatural about that.

AUGUST

Vibrating in a Material World

Thanks to recent innovations in technology, we've come a long way from the cheap, hard plastic vibrators of the past. But even the most intrepid pleasure shopper may be flummoxed by the variety of materials on the market today. Here's a brief guide:

+ **Silicone:** Used to make high-quality vibrators and vibrator sleeves that are non-porous and easy to clean. Expensive, but probably worth the extra cost.

+ **Cyberskin:** Soft and pliable, cyberskin is a recent innovation that feels more like real skin than anything on the market. It's very porous, so use it with a condom or clean it carefully after each use.

+ **Rubber:** Easy to find and inexpensive, synthetic rubber vibrators are soft and warm, but may not last as long as more expensive types.

+ **Plastic:** Vinyl and soft plastic toys are inexpensive and lightweight, but porous. Hard plastic vibrators are non-porous, making them easier to clean, but they may not last that long.

+ **Soft acrylic:** Another soft, non-porous material that can be found on toys like the head of the Hitachi Magic Wand.

+ **Natural rubber latex:** Used most often for condoms and gloves, this material is occasionally used in sex toys. It is incompatible with any kind of oil.

Remember that any porous material requires the use of a condom and careful cleaning after play. In fact, it's a good idea to clean any toy after use, and store it afterwards in a cool, dry place. With a little care, your vibrator will be buzzing happily for a long time.

AUGUST

Welcoming a Backdoor Guest

If you're interested in exploring anal penetration, the keys to a pleasurable experience are communication, relaxation, and lubrication. Be clear with your partner about your expectations, and spend some time getting comfortable before you dive in. At the very least, ask him to massage your buttocks, which will stimulate the general area. You may even want to have an orgasm to further relax you. When you're ready to move on, the most important thing to remember is lubrication, and lots of it, because this area is not self-lubricating. Apply lube not only to his condom-covered penis but all around your anal opening and even inside it.

Then, have him start by slowly penetrating you with one, then possibly two, lubed fingers. Once your anus is relaxed, he can hold the tip of his penis at your opening. Breathe deeply from your belly, then bear down on his member. Remember, the person being penetrated—in this case, that's you—sets the pace. Ask him to move in and then stop before continuing as you get used to the sensation. If it hurts, stop. He should aim for your belly button first, then, after he's touched the first curve of your rectum, aim toward your backbone. Wait until he's completely in before letting hands roam to your nipples or clit: Stimulating other erogenous zones could cause an involuntary contraction of your sphincter and push him out.

Once he's thrusting gently, pull his hand around to massage your other tender parts. "The hottest thing a lover's ever done for me is give me anal sex while rubbing my vaginal area," says Liane, a doctor in her early forties. "We ended up coming together!"

AUGUST

Toys for Backdoor Play

Toys made especially for your behind make both partner sex and solo explorations lots of fun. Butt plugs, for example, are essentially short dildos with flared bases that prevent them from getting lost inside you. (Don't put anything that *doesn't* have a flared base up your derriere.) Plugs come in a variety of sizes, shapes, and materials. Look for soft jelly rubber when you're starting out; it's porous, so you'll definitely want to use a condom.

Most plugs have a narrow tip and a wide body that then narrows again before the base. Once you slip the plug inside, your body closes around the narrow neck, holding the plug in place while you carry on. (If you plan to do any thrusting, look for a long, slim version.) To enjoy the lusty sensations of double penetration, try pleasuring yourself with your favorite vibrator—or your man—while wearing a plug. Remember that rectal tissue is very thin and doesn't self-lubricate, so don't scrimp on the lube. Use lots and lots—and then some more.

A string of marble-sized anal beads makes another exotic backdoor toy. Many people love the sensation of their muscles opening and closing around each bead; others just find it distracting. Some people intensify their climax or their partner's by gently pulling out the beads one by one as they achieve an orgasm. Check with your partner before trying this, and don't yank!

A word about materials: Cheaply-made plastic anal beads often have rough, sharp seams, but it's nothing a little attention with a nail file can't fix. Rubber beads are softer, but porous, so slip a condom over them and knot it at the end. And silicone beads—well, they're expensive, but sometimes your pleasure deserves the very best.

AUGUST

Give Him a Signal

Good foreplay starts long before you even enter the bedroom. Showing your man how much you want him, when there's little or no way to consummate your lust, builds anticipation for the moment when you *are* finally alone. So find a way to signal your intentions to him with a sultry look or a delicate touch. Develop a specific, secret sign that you can use when you're out in public to tell each other "Let's get out of here so I can rip your clothes off and ravish you."

You can use your secret signals at home, too. One friend of mine tells me that because her teenage son would be "totally grossed out" by overt displays of affection between his parents, she and her husband give each other surreptitious touches and pats while they're making dinner and going about their evening. Not only does this signal to each other that they're both in the mood, but it heightens their excitement. "We can hardly wait to go to bed!" she says.

You can also communicate your interest by setting the mood in your bedroom. Michelle, a thirty-three-year-old corporate trainer, suggests keeping candles in the bedroom. "When you're in the mood and your significant other is getting ready for bed, you can quickly light the candles, get naked, and be ready to show your interest!"

HISTORICAL NOTE: Today is the birthday of Madonna (1958-), American singer and sexual icon.

AUGUST

"I used to be Snow White…but I drifted."
—Mae West (1892-1980)

Happy Birthday, Mae West!

Born on this day in Brooklyn, New York, American icon Mae West was known for her portrayals of sexy, emancipated women and scorn for conventional morality. Have you ever daydreamed about being as unabashedly outspoken as West or modern icons like Madonna? Why not indulge in a little role-playing for one evening? Taking on a different role, even temporarily, can be enormously freeing—not to mention fun! Here are some ideas for stepping outside your everyday persona:

✦ Go to a bar or party separately. Flirt with your partner outrageously. Recapture the delicious, naughty fun of "picking up" each other.

✦ Rent a hotel room, and have him go there first. Show up at the hotel door wearing nothing underneath. Or you go to the room first, and order up a handsome stud (him)!

✦ In the privacy of your own home, enact a secret fantasy—but tonight, in honor of Mae West, you're the one in charge. Play at being mistress/slave, teacher/student, lady cop/prisoner.

The key to fun when role-playing is making sure that the rules are clear at the outset. To keep the erotic charge, stay in character throughout the game, but be sure to have a "safe word" either of you can use to mean "stop right now!" The safe word must be obeyed immediately and without question. Never force your partner to do anything he doesn't want to do. With a few simple ground rules, you can make sure your evening of "being bad" is very good!

AUGUST

Position of the Week: Seagulls on the Wing

The *T'ung Hsüan Tzu* by Li T'ung Hsüan delights in describing sexual positions with highly evocative language that often references the beauty of nature. Seagulls on the Wing is one such posture. It closely resembles the Ninth Posture of *The Perfumed Garden* (see July 15), only here, instead of lying on your stomach as he enters you from behind, you're lying on your back with your hips at the edge of the bed. Place your feet on the floor as he kneels in front of you. Instead of slanting down into you, his member will enter directly into you, resulting in some interesting sensations. Abandon yourself to erotic pleasure as he thrusts away. Your clitoris will be more accessible than it is in a conventional missionary position, because you won't have to worry about sliding a hand between your bodies. Take advantage of it by stroking yourself with a vibrator or your fingers, or guide his hands to your anxiously awaiting love button.

You can adapt this position for use in any room of the house. On a hot summer's day, imagine lying at the edge of a swimming pool as he swan dives into you.

AUGUST

More Booty for Your Booty

If a clitoris or vagina gets turned on by vibration, why wouldn't the millions of nerve endings around your anus? Some butt plugs come with battery packs; others have hollow shafts into which you can slip a battery vibe. There are also long, thin probes that vibrate and rotate!

But don't think you have to go on a shopping spree. Many vibrators come with anal attachments to turn them into vibrating butt plugs. If yours doesn't have a cord, make sure it's long enough that you can keep a grip on it, even in the heat of passion. Larger vibrators can be adapted with flexible anal "sleeves," although I'd skip the fringes and nubs offered by many novelty makers. Keep it simple.

Give your open-minded man a thrill by circling and dipping the tip of your well-lubed vibrator into his anus during intercourse or manual or oral sex. He's just as sensitive down there as you are! G-spot vibrators can even do double-duty as prostate stimulators. Just remember to never put anything that's been in someone's derriere into your vagina without changing the condom first. Or better yet, buy him his own set of toys! Despite what Mom says, sometimes it's okay not to share.

AUGUST

Awakening the Fifth Chakra

Have you ever heard someone say that they tried to speak, but "the words caught in my throat?" Tantrists would say that this person has a blocked fifth—or throat—chakra. This energy center governs communication, including our creativity and our ability to express ourselves. Blocks here result from repressing our ideas and feelings, which can ruin relationships and make satisfying sex impossible. To awaken a blocked throat chakra, find safe ways to express yourself. Sing, chant, or hum when you're alone or in the car. Learn how to breathe consciously, find a class in pranayama in your area, or keep a journal in which you can explore your innermost thoughts and feelings.

With your lover, work to communicate more openly and intimately. Don't lie and say you enjoy things you don't—and never fake an orgasm—and don't expect your lover to have ESP. Here's a great exercise suggested to me by a very wise therapist: Each of you "reserve" an hour of the other's time on different nights of the week. During your hour, go into the bedroom and get comfortable. The person whose hour it is gets say how it's spent—cuddling, making out, or just talking—with one exception: *You can't have intercourse.* You'll be amazed at how much closer you'll feel after a quiet hour of sharing your respective days as you rub each other's feet.

Open communication is difficult, but it's perhaps the most intimate thing you can do. Expressing tough emotions can be a tremendous relief, in the end, you'll feel not only closer to your lover, but closer to yourself.

AUGUST

Anchors Away!

Do you live near water? Making love on a boat, with the waves slapping gently on the hull in time to your thrusts, beats a waterbed anytime. If you're lucky enough to own a sailboat or powerboat, head out to the middle of a bay or a lake for your own personal pleasure cruise. Cut the engine, lower the sails, and drop anchor. Head below deck or simply keep close to the center of the boat, which offers the most stability. (Safety note: If your boat is small or you're on deck under the stars, it's a good idea to keep your life jackets on!) In smaller boats, lay some cushions down.

On a hot summer day, float down a lazy river on a rubber raft. You may not be able to have actual intercourse, but there's no reason that your hands can't get busy. Demonstrate some of the manual or oral moves you've learned this year, and he'll be yelling "Thar he blows!" before too long. Afterwards, drop over the side for a post-orgasm wake-up dip.

If you can't get access to any aquatic vessels, there's always the beach. On a clear night, lay out a towel and roll around in time to the pounding of the surf. (Have an extra towel on hand in case you need to cover up quickly.) And don't worry about a little sand—that's what showers are for!

AUGUST

Ice, Ice Baby

One of the best sexual toys is right in your freezer: Ice can be used to create a variety of thrilling sensations on any part of the body, especially on a steamy summer day. Try rubbing an ice cube over his nipples. Trail it down over his back or stomach to his most sensitive regions. Hold an ice cube in your mouth while you go down on him. The contrast between your warm mouth and the cold ice will send him over the edge. Or alternate between sliding the ice along his shaft and pleasuring him with your hot mouth. Or try a combo platter. My friend Lee, a forty-year-old researcher, advises, "Ice his balls before giving him oral sex. The contrast makes the area very sensitive."

Ice can be fun for you, too. Stroke an ice cube across your nipples, and watch them become rock hard, or slip a cube between your lower lips, and over your clitoris and vaginal opening, imagining the hot friction of his penis inside you. Along these lines, my friend Kyle suggests freezing a dildo wrapped in plastic wrap or a condom, and using the sensation of the frozen toy against your hot skin to drive yourself wild. Try a chilled cucumber or water-filled condom for your own foray into the wonderful world of ice sculpture.

AUGUST

Virgo, the Virgin

If your or your man's birthday falls between today and September 22, then you were born under the sun sign of Virgo, symbolized by a virgin. According to astrologers, Virgos are practical, no-nonsense, hard-working types with a strong perfectionist streak. Although they can be critical, know that they are equally critical of themselves—if not more so. They're deeply concerned with health and order, so make sure you take care of yourself and keep the clutter in your home to a minimum. Your Virgo likes his surroundings tidy and his person well groomed.

Virgos aren't known for their wild spontaneity when it comes to sex, so your best bet at seducing your Virgo is by moving slowly. Work on building trust between the two of you (if you're a Virgo yourself, know that you'll need to trust a man to bed him). Be open and honest in your attraction to him, and appeal to his intellectual and health-conscious nature by stressing the many benefits of sexual activity. Pack a picnic basket full of organic foods and plan a sexy *al fresco* picnic. If you rehearse some of the moves together beforehand and pick your spot carefully, you'll reduce his anxiety about doing something so daring.

If you're a Virgo yourself, see if you can't manage your perfectionism. Remember that sex is messy—and if you must take a shower before lovemaking, invite your lover to join you. Sex is also supposed to be fun, so try to give your Inner Schoolmarm the day off. Challenge your man to a kid's game, updated for adults. Think how much fun a game of tag would be—in the nude!

AUGUST

Strike a Pose

Dreading the endless parade of summer vacation pictures from friends and family? Customize this annual tradition by creating a naughty album for your eyes and his only. It's a great way to unleash any exhibitionist streaks, and you can be as elaborate or as risqué as you like. Ask a photographer friend to help you with a surprise album for your man that captures you in a variety of sultry poses; in return, let him use the best ones for his portfolio. By the way, a photographer friend who has shot photos of nude models tells me he's too busy arranging the shot to get excited by a bared breast or buttock. A professional will put you at ease and photograph you in ways that make you proud of your body.

However, in these days of digital cameras, you don't have to go the professional route. Using your camera's timer, take an erotic photo of yourself and leave it somewhere only he will find it. Take pictures of each other or of both of you together, and look at them whenever you want to get your motors running. Just be sure you delete your camera work after you're done with your modeling session, or hide the results in a file to which only you have access.

AUGUST

Position of the Week: The Swing

Remember those wonderful summer days of childhood, and the feeling of flying back and forth on a park swing, higher and higher into the air? Later, as we grew older, we might have enjoyed gently rocking back and forth on a porch swing with our sweetheart. Well, you can turn your bed into a playground, according to the *Kama Sutra*! Just try the charming position that Vatsyayana describes as The Swing. While you may not fly above the ground, you'll definitely feel like you're soaring.

Ask your man to lean back onto his hands. He can also lie back on some big overstuffed pillows. Then, facing his feet, lower yourself down onto his waiting erection, your thighs straddling his. Tilt your body forward and grasp his shins. This will give you the balance you need to rock your pelvis gently back and forward. If you're shy about touching yourself in front of him, this position allows you to stroke your nub without him seeing—although chances are that he'll know and be titillated by your growing excitement, as well as the sight of your derriere bumping on top of him. Let his thrusts push you higher and higher!

AUGUST

Entering by His Backdoor

Many heterosexual men find the experience of anal penetration to be a huge turn-on. And why shouldn't they? As we've discussed elsewhere, the anus is chock-full of nerve endings, and anal penetration stimulates both the bulb of his penis and his prostate gland (a.k.a. the male G-spot). Enjoying it doesn't mean he's gay. Again, remember that sexuality is defined by *whom* you have sex with, not how. Lots of gay men have never had anal intercourse, whereas many straight couples love it—as the popularity of the *Bend Over Boyfriend* series of videos indicates.

If your man wants to explore anal penetration, the process is pretty much the same as it is for you (see August 14). Start by massaging his anus with a well-lubed, well-manicured finger; putting a condom or latex glove on your hand isn't a bad idea, because it will feel smoother. When he's relaxed enough to accommodate two of your fingers, you can graduate to a well-lubed dildo or a toy designed especially for the anus. Again, use *lots* of lube, and check in with him frequently. Remember that throughout the experience, he should set the pace.

When he's ready, put the dildo against his anus and let him bear down on it as he inhales and exhales. Don't be surprised if he loses his erection as he adjusts to the feeling. When he gives you the okay, you can start moving inside him. Experiment with different positions— rear entry gives you the best chance of hitting his prostate, but you can basically use any position you use for vaginal intercourse. If he wants you to, stroke his nipples or penis, and when you're done, a good backdoor guest exits *slowly*, so that his muscles don't tense up. Afterwards, cuddle!

AUGUST

Electrifying Oral Sex

Your favorite vibrator can turn great oral sex into fantastic oral sex. Ask him to start off by humming as he sucks and licks your clitoris. The sound vibrations can feel divine. If he doesn't want you to know that he can't carry a tune, assure him that his moans of excitement will have the same effect. Then bring it up a notch by having him put a vibrator under his tongue as he caresses you. *Voilà*—supercharged oral sex! By the way, make sure he feels free to use the vibrator elsewhere—around or in your vaginal opening or anus—as he pleasures you with his tongue, as long as it doesn't distract you.

When it's his turn to enjoy your oral skills, your trusty vibrator can come in handy. Hold your vibrator against the base of his penis or his testicles. Press it to his perineum. Circle it around his anus. Some men even like to be anally penetrated by a vibrator or dildo during oral sex. Look for a vibrator designed for G-spot or prostate stimulation, or a vibrating butt plug.

If he finds that a vibrator distracts him from the wonderful things you're doing with your mouth, there's no reason why you can't use your toy to pleasure yourself while you're pleasuring him (as long as you can keep your focus on your oral technique). Imagine how electrifying it would be if you came together!

AUGUST

It's Okay to Point

How can you show your man that you'd like him to worship your love button with his mouth? If you're too shy to tell him verbally, or you just want to try something different, try the "point and kiss" game. Tell him that you want him to kiss you wherever you point. Start with your lips, and move down your body bit by bit. Point to your neck, your breasts, your nipples, and your belly button. Then work your way down to your pubic hair and the spot where your labia meet. By this point, he'll have gotten the point, so to speak.

Now that you've shown him what you want, show him your appreciation! If he's doing it right, moan your arousal; if he needs some pointers, now's the time to whisper some breathy and encouraging instructions, along the lines of "Oooohhhh, I love it when you flick it from side-to-side." Run your fingers through his hair. Suck on one of *his* fingers. Let him see how much you're enjoying yourself.

Another move that men find extremely sexy is when you reach down to hold your love lips open while they're pleasuring you. The sight is incredibly erotic for him, and by pulling the skin taut, you increase your own sensations. You can also do this while he watches you pleasure yourself.

AUGUST

Summer Camp for Adults

Many of us look forward to Labor Day weekend, the last holiday and long weekend of the summer, so why not take advantage of the weather to plan a little camping trip with your man? Reserve a campsite at a national park, or sign up for a backpacking or river-rafting trip. At night, zip your sleeping bags together, and make love under the stars or by a roaring campfire (or just raise the temperature inside your tent!). If you can find a campsite near a river, you'll enjoy your lovemaking accompanied by the sound of rushing water.

My friend Harry, a thirty-seven-year-old director, comments that "I find that there's something about isolating yourself together in an environment of natural beauty that does the trick as far as firing up my libido. I think we're very tied to nature instinctively, but we're so caught up in the stress and worry of our daily urban lives that we literally can lose touch with our sexual selves. A city guy taken into a secluded natural setting with his lover will have a lot more libido." Don't be surprised if your weekend in the Great Outdoors unleashes your man's animal instincts!

AUGUST

Love Your Body!

To many women, summer means bathing suits, and bathing suits mean utter dread. What a tragedy! While it's great to be healthy and fit, too many of us compare ourselves to the unattainable (and often unhealthy) standards of physical beauty promoted by the media. Somehow, we've gotten the message that we don't deserve—and won't have—wonderful sex unless our bodies are "perfect" by some stranger's standards.

As a result, some women don't enjoy the full range of sexual pleasure to which they're entitled simply because they're afraid of their man seeing them naked. As my friend Melissa puts it, "In this image-conscious world, so many women hold back on their sexuality, waiting until they've lost that five or ten pounds. My attitude is that no matter what your size or weight, you should live, love, and screw! A woman with a healthy sexual appetite is much more arousing to a man than a repressed stick figure."

So if you really want to achieve sensual ecstasy every day, learn to love your body. Don't fill it with junk, but don't beat yourself up if you don't look like the anorexic models in *Vogue.* Yes, exercise will improve your health, which will make you feel more energetic and thus sexier, but that doesn't mean you have to spend hours in the gym to have a great sex life. Appreciate your body for all the wonderful sensations it provides. Indulge your five senses. Adorn yourself in your favorite perfumes. Learn to give and receive massages. Wear clothing that makes you feel fabulous. Have lots and lots of delicious orgasms.

And if you don't like how you look in a bathing suit—skinny dip!

AUGUST

Have a Great (Manual) Labor Day

Labor Day falls on a different Monday in September every year, so the following list of preview tips will help you make the most of this last summer holiday. You work hard throughout the year, but today we'll talk about some manual-labor techniques that are more enjoyable than back-breaking. Here are some techniques for your man to try on you:

+ With his hand cupped to form the letter C, he slides his thumb into your vagina and rocks his hand so that his thumb presses on your G-spot while his fingers massage your clitoris and love lips.

+ Have him spread your labia with the fingers of one hand. His other hand goes on top, where his middle finger can stroke your button.

+ This one's easiest if he's lying next to you or spooning into you. He curves three fingers over your mons so that his middle finger can stroke your clitoris in whatever way you like best, while his index and ring fingers massage your lips.

+ While he's lying next to you, have him slide one hand under your butt as his top hand pleasures you from above. The fingers of the lower hand can caress your derrière, play with your rosebud, slip into your vagina—or all of the above.

Have fun with these techniques. If they work, great; if not, there's nothing wrong with your tried-and-true approach. After all, sex is supposed to be fun—not work!

CHAPTER NINE

SEPTEMBER

"It is only the ignorant who despise education."
—Publilius Syrus, Roman writer, first century B.C.

Educate yourself—sexually!

Like many people, you may associate September with the end of the long, lazy days of summer vacation. With a heavy heart, you bid goodbye to warm evenings and relaxing vacations. If you've got kids, you may be dealing with back-to-school stress. So why not further *your* education—your sexual education? This month's tips will use September as a time to explore new positions and techniques, and learn fun sexual trivia. Tips will highlight information from sex how-to manuals from around the world giving new meaning to the term "teacher's pet."

This month's birth flowers are *aster* and *morning glory*. In Victorian times, an aster had several different meanings, including a love of variety, or daintiness, while the morning glory symbolized affection. Appropriate these flowers for your own meanings: A bouquet of asters might encourage you to explore a variety of sexual techniques and positions, while a morning glory might remind you to be true to yourself.

The ancient Greeks used this month's birthstone, the *sapphire*, to stimulate the opening of the third eye and to tap into the subconscious. The guardian of love, the sapphire was given to one's sweetheart to enhance love, banish envy and jealousy, and ensure fidelity.

SEPTEMBER

Sex: Just What the Doctor Ordered

Sex isn't just good for your genitals: It's good for every part of your body, as today's researchers are discovering. One hot area of study is the hormone oxytocin. During an orgasm, blood levels of oxytocin—known as the "cuddle hormone" because of its role in helping us form emotional bonds—surge up to five times their normal levels. Because oxytocin regulates functions such as temperature, blood pressure, and the healing of wounds, experts are focusing on its role in the relationship between sex and health. Here are some other benefits that scientists are exploring:

+ **It's good for your heart.** Not only is sex great aerobic exercise, but studies also indicate that sexually active people have fewer heart attacks. Sex hormones DHEA and testosterone may also reduce the risk of heart disease.

+ **It can help you lose weight.** Each act of intercourse burns about 200 calories, equivalent to half an hour of running. Which would you rather do?

+ **It controls pain.** Orgasms release endorphins and corticosteroids, temporarily relieving the pain of menstrual cramps, arthritis, and migraines.

+ **It boosts immunity.** Frequent sex may boost levels of infection-fighting antibodies, and help your body heal wounds.

+ **It may fight cancer.** Studies are trying to determine whether sex hormones prevent cancerous cells from developing, lowering the risk of breast and prostate cancer.

+ **It improves your mental health.** Hormones released during sexual activity help calm anxiety, ease fear, and relieve depression.

Researchers are even studying the links between frequent orgasms and longevity. One study in Scotland indicated that sex actually slows the aging process. Stay tuned! In the meantime, it appears that an orgasm a day may very well keep the doctor away.

SEPTEMBER

Position of the Week: Fitting on of the Sock

Even in the male-dominated North African culture of the late fifteenth century, erotic texts such as *The Perfumed Garden* by Sheikh Nefzawi stressed the importance of foreplay to a woman's pleasure:

"If you would have pleasant coition, which ought to give an equal share of happiness to the two combatants and be satisfactory to both, you must first of all toy with the woman, excite her with kisses, by nibbling and sucking her lips, by caressing her neck and cheeks…If you have done as I said, the enjoyment will come to both of you simultaneously. This it is which makes the pleasure of the woman so sweet."

To this end, the Fitting on of the Sock is not so much a position as a technique to get you all hot and bothered. Essentially, he uses his penis as a dildo. You lie on your back and he kneels between your legs, placing his member between your love lips, which he pulls gently closed around him with his thumb and index finger. He then rubs your entire vulva, including your clitoris, with the tip of his penis, giving you "a lively rubbing" until you're wet from his secretions and your own love juices. When you're "amply prepared for enjoyment" by the movement of his "weapon" in your "scabbard," he can thrust in you to the hilt.

SEPTEMBER

Ready, Set, Go! A Quick Course on Quickies

Long, tender lovemaking sessions are wonderful, but there's nothing like the exhilaration of spur-of-the-moment sex. Not only is it a great mood-lifter, but it also keeps the flames burning by showing him that you have to have him *right here, right now.* There's nothing like a little fast nooky to break up the monotony of any chore. (You're folding laundry together when suddenly boom! You're *on* the laundry.) Studies have shown that couples who speed up sex once in a while actually have sex more often—and that they cuddle and kiss more, too.

Here are some tips for making your super-fast session all that it can be. First, you should both be up for spontaneous sex. Ambushing your partner—catching him at an inopportune or inappropriate moment, like the last thirty seconds of a playoff game—may have the opposite effect from what you intended. Also, by its very nature, a quickie precludes extensive foreplay, so it may be work best when you're already aroused: You've been talking about sex; you've been having the mother of all makeout sessions; you're looking at Internet porn together half an hour before you're supposed to be at the in-laws. If not, use a little lube or saliva (and your own hands) to move things along.

So be a little late for lunch. You'll both feel great!

SEPTEMBER

A Primer on Going Public

Many people fantasize about having sex in a public place, and the thrill of getting caught only heightens their arousal—no doubt because fear causes the body to produce adrenaline, the same chemical your body makes when you're horny. Remember, sex in public is illegal (see May 1), so use your discretion. Your best bet is the cover of night, when there are fewer people around. When outdoors, pick concealed spots where you can see people approaching: on or between parked cars, on top of a building, in an enclosed balcony or backyard, or on a remote beach. When indoors, look for rooms with doors you can lock, like an office or closet. Elevators aren't good for much besides foreplay: Many have closed-circuit cameras. More importantly, you won't have time to do much between floors.

No matter where you are, the longer you take, the greater your chances of being discovered. Only attempt public sex with a partner whose body and responses you know well. Underwear is an obstacle, so don't wear it unless it's a G-string or thong that can be easily pushed aside. A long skirt can be hiked up to provide easy access.

Standing positions—you leaning over so he can enter you from behind, or sitting on a horizontal surface like a wall or table—are easiest to recover from if someone approaches. Never attempt public sex if you're under the influence of drugs or alcohol. If you're going public, you need to keep your wits about you!

SEPTEMBER

Deep Throating

First made famous by the 1972 Linda Lovelace movie *Deep Throat*, deep throating refers to the practice of taking his entire penis into your mouth and throat. You won't be able to suck or lick or do much with your tongue, so this trick is more impressive than practical. The key is positioning: You've got to widen the angle of your mouth and throat into a straight line. That's why the most common position for deep throating is lying on your back with your head hanging off the edge of the bed while your man kneels or stands in front of you, his penis at mouth level. You can also sit on his chest, facing his feet and shaft. If you don't think you'll get distracted, you can even assume the 69 position.

Your throat's natural reaction to having something blocking it will be to gag. Relax, and remember to breathe through your nose. Keep your hands at the base of his penis to push him out if you need to, or control his thrusts by putting your hands on his thighs. If you're concerned that you'll gag if he comes in your throat, have him wear a condom.

Deep throating takes practice and a relaxed attitude. If it's not for you, don't sweat it. You can blow a pretty impressive tune without his flute getting anywhere near your tonsils.

SEPTEMBER

Mouthwork Positions for Advanced Students

Don't think that the only position for cunnilingus is with him between your legs, his feet dangling off the edge of the bed. Here are some other positions to try:

+ Keep your legs together. This works well if your super-sensitive love button can't handle a full-on assault.

+ Try a modified sixty-nine: He lies next to you facing your feet, with his hips by your head and shoulders and his upper torso lying across your hips. This allows him to approach your clitoris with a downward stroke, and gives his neck a nice break.

+ When he's between your legs, drape one leg over his shoulder and twist slightly. This gives him even better access to your sweet spot.

EXTRA CREDIT: The best way to describe this position is as an upward sixty-nine. He's sitting up on a couch, his hips at the edge of the cushion. You crawl onto him *carefully* with your thighs on his shoulders, your feet clasping behind his head. (Yes, you're upside down.) Your shoulders and upper arms rest on his thighs. He holds you *tightly* as he pleasures you. You'll get an interesting blood rush to your brain, but you'll probably want to use this as a transition to horizontal positions.

SEPTEMBER

Teach Him the ABCs

In one of his profane, hilarious routines, the late comedian Sam Kinison dispensed an invaluable bit of advice to men on how to perform oral sex on women: Lick the alphabet! That's right: All your man has to do is draw the letters of the alphabet on your clitoris with his tongue. Heck, he can move on to composing love letters and sonnets on your button if he wants.

This a great way to get your man to realize that you don't necessarily need wild flicking, but gentle, subtle pressure that allows your arousal to build to fever pitch—something great lovers learn. "My fiancé gives the most amazing oral sex," says Karen, an English teacher in her twenties. "I don't know what he does, but he goes in mini-rounds, licking for awhile and then stopping and doing something else and then going back to licking. It's wild and creates the most fabulous orgasms."

The best thing about the alphabet technique is that he can practice it any time. Suggest that he hold a breath mint or candy against his teeth (LifeSavers work great) and trace its ridges, curves and holes with the tip of his tongue. You can even do this together: It certainly won't hurt you to work on your tongue dexterity. No one has to know what you're doing. What a way to liven up a boring meeting!

SEPTEMBER

Never Fake an Orgasm

When it comes to absolutes about issues other than practicing safe sex, there's one biggie: Never fake an orgasm. Let's face it, you're doing the two of you a great disservice. First of all, there's a good chance he can tell: It's pretty hard (read: impossible) to fake the involuntary 0.8-second orgasmic contractions of your PC muscle. Second, you'll trap yourself in a cycle of deceit that will almost ensure that you'll *never* get what you need. It's pretty hard to stop someone in the middle of what they think you love and announce, "You know, that never really worked for me."

And why would you want to fake an orgasm? Are you afraid your lover will think he isn't doing a good job? Well, maybe he isn't, because maybe you haven't told him or shown him what you need! Or maybe you fake it because you know you're not going to come. Don't buy into the unrealistic expectation that you have to have an orgasm every time. A loving "It's not going to happen for me tonight, honey, I'm too stressed/tired/whatever," takes the pressure off both of you and is infinitely better than a lie. Reassure him, profusely, and, if it's true, tell him how much you enjoyed the rest of the encounter. If you're open with him, you'll feel safer, and if you feel safer, the chances of you climaxing next time are much, much greater.

If, heaven forbid, you have been faking, start asking him to do more of what you *do* like. Suggest trying some of the techniques in this book, and if he wants to know why the "old" technique isn't working, tell him your body's changing. It's true: You now know what it needs.

SEPTEMBER

Position of the Week: The Intact Posture

Composed during an age where premarital and extramarital sex were common, the *Kama Sutra* was written for all lovers, women as well as men. The *Ananga Ranga* of the late fifteenth century is the product of a very different society: Its audience is married men, to whom Kalyana Malla offers specific instruction for pleasing their spouses sexually, in order to prevent the boredom that can creep into any long-term relationship. "This book is composed," he writes, "with the object of preventing lives and loves being wasted," a goal as worthy today as it was five hundred years ago.

Malla viewed the various forms of sexual congress as an art, giving them detailed descriptions and poetic names. The reclining position that Malla calls the Intact Posture appears to be named as such because the woman is folded up like a little intact package. Lie on your back and bend your knees deeply, resting your shins or feet against your man's chest as he enters you from a kneeling position, "and embraces and enjoys" you. To make penetration easier, he can slide his hands under your buttocks to lift you onto his thighs. Once he's inside, use your hands—or his—to stroke and fondle your breasts and clitoris. Your range of movement will be limited, so make good use of that PC muscle!

SEPTEMBER

Self-Loving Reason #9: Frustration Begone!

It would be nice if we always wanted to make love when our partners wanted to, but that just isn't the way real life is. Given the natural ebb and flow of energy desire, it's unrealistic to expect that our libidos will always be perfectly in sync with the object of our lust. Both men and women have their cycles. Some days you feel about as sexy as a wet rag and he's raring to go; other times, he'll be the one who's too stressed out for amorous adventures, while you're five minutes away from humping his leg.

Masturbation, however, is the great equalizer. Knowing that you can take care of business yourself relieves the strain on both of you. Why pressure someone who's not in the mood if you've got your five fingers? A loving partner won't begrudge you a little release because God knows, it will be his turn one day. Watching you may even change his mind.

Self-loving also comes in handy, no pun intended, when you're single or your partner isn't around. Think you're just going to pass out from frustration while he's on that business trip? No need! You can pleasure yourself any time of the day, and almost anywhere. Relief and ecstasy are right at your fingertips.

SEPTEMBER

Let Him Teach You

The best information about how to please your man won't come from a book—it will come from him. Every man has a different masturbation technique, and unless you have ESP, you're not going to know what it is unless you watch and learn. "The best thing you can do is learn how your guy likes to be brought off," advises my friend Kyle. "Masturbating feels good to him, but letting your hand do the same thing is fantastic. Have him show you what he does, and then try it to mimic it. Don't feel criticized if he tells you to go harder or faster. Encourage him to give you feedback."

What if he's shy about masturbating in front of you? Many people have been conditioned to feel shame about self-pleasuring. He may even feel embarrassed to admit that he masturbates without you. (By the way, a man's solo pleasuring is more about physical release than sex; many happily coupled men masturbate regularly.) Reassure him that you find watching him incredibly hot. Show your interest. Ask him questions. When it's your turn, have him guide your hand.

When you watch him masturbate, you'll notice things about his sexual response that you might miss if you were actively involved: The way his chest flushes, the veins that stand out on his neck, his rapid breathing, the position of his fingers. This is one time where it definitely pays to be an "A-plus" voyeur.

HISTORICAL NOTE: Today is the birthday of D.H. Lawrence (1885-1930), the English writer whose novel *Lady Chatterley's Lover* wasn't published in England until thirty years after his death.

SEPTEMBER

Safer Sex Seminar

Fear not, this is by no means a lecture, just a simple review of facts. From having read earlier months, you may already know that one in five people in the United States have had a sexually transmitted disease (STD). You also can't tell if someone has an STD by looking at them. In fact, eighty percent of the population has been exposed to genital warts. It's also been estimated that one in five people have genital herpes—but eighty percent don't know it. Taking all that into consideration, it's time to discuss the many fun benefits of practicing safer sex:

+ It gives you peace of mind, allowing you to enjoy sex more.

+ It shows respect for the sexual health of yourself and your partner, which makes everyone feel good.

+ Condoms can help him stay hard longer, meaning more fun for everyone.

+ Condoms make for quick post-nooky cleanup, and help keep your sex toys clean as well.

+ In combination with lube, latex barriers like condoms and dental dams can provide interesting sensations to both partners.

+ Latex barriers allow you to try practices like oral-anal stimulation (a.k.a. analingus or "rimming") without worrying about hygiene or sexual fluids.

+ Safe sex practices encourage you to be creative and communicate about sex, promoting deeper intimacy.

So instead of moping about how condoms and other latex barriers are such a drag, think of them as "get-out-of-jail-free" cards ("jail" being an incurable STD) that open up a whole new world of sensual creativity, bring you closer to your partner, and enable you to enjoy erotic bliss worry-free. Class dismissed!

SEPTEMBER

Be a Smart Condom Shopper

Throughout their long and colorful history, condoms have been made from almost every material imaginable, including seedpods, linen, oiled silk paper, papyrus soaked in water, and even fish bladders. Luckily, today you have several materials from which to choose when picking out your prophylactic:

+ **Latex.** Latex condoms have several things going for them: They're cheap, convenient, and highly effective (if used correctly) against STDs and pregnancy. Disadvantages: They're incompatible with oil-based lubes and prone to breakage if used incorrectly, and some people are allergic to them.

+ **Polyurethane.** A recent innovation, polyurethane condoms are the wunderkinds of condomland. Polyurethane is thinner than latex, transparent, odor-free, and tasteless. It's hypoallergenic; transmits heat better (so he'll feel more); isn't as sensitive to heat and light; and is compatible with oil-based lubricants. However, the FDA hasn't officially approved polyurethane for STD prevention or contraception, even though studies show that sperm and viruses can't pass through it. Polyurethane isn't as elastic as latex, either, so it may break if used without lube or incorrectly.

+ **Lambskin.** These condoms, made from sheep intestines, may feel more natural and may work for contraception, but viruses like HIV can permeate them, so they are definitely not recommended for safer sex.

Where's the best place to buy condoms? While most drugstores today carry a fairly large assortment, go online to sites like Affordable-Condoms.com, Condomania.com, Condom.com, CondomZone.com and SafeSex.com for an even larger selection. Shop around for the best prices!

SEPTEMBER

Make Your Condom-Shopping Checklist

The next time your man gives you that tired old line that wearing a rubber is like wearing a raincoat, point out that raincoats don't come in as many sizes, styles, colors, textures, and flavors:

+ **Size.** "Large" often refers to diameter, not length. You definitely don't want a condom that's too small, because it will break more easily, slip off, leave too much skin exposed, and just be darned uncomfortable. Too large, and… well, you've got troubles.

+ **Texture.** There are condoms that feature little nubs on the inside, on the outside (ostensibly for your pleasure), and both.

+ **Flavors.** Latex condoms come in flavors ranging from strawberry and chocolate to mint and even cola, which is a nice addition to oral sex. Since oils won't hurt polyurethane condoms, dress these up with treats like chocolate and whipped cream, or products made for this purpose.

+ **Color.** Good for folks with a sense of humor. There's even a glow-in-the-dark condom.

+ **Lubricated.** These are coated with either water-based or silicone-based lube. If contraception is your main concern, choose one with a spermicide like nonoxynol-9. Otherwise, pick a non-lubricated variety (nonoxynol-9 can irritate the vagina, which can spread infection) and add lube yourself.

But wait, there's more! Do you want a balloon top? A condom that covers the testicles? Other special features? Read the box. Check the label, too, to see whether the FDA has approved your brand for STD prevention or contraception. Shop smart, and love well!

HISTORICAL NOTE: Today is the birthday of Margaret Sanger (1883-1996), American pioneer of the birth control movement.

SEPTEMBER

Prophylactic Protocol

Having grown up in the age of AIDS, many younger men simply consider condom use part of the action, so you won't need to do much convincing. But if a prospective lover refuses to wear a condom, you might seriously reconsider whether you really want him as a bedmate. His attitude shows a stunning lack of consideration for his health and yours. If your man says he doesn't like condoms, ask him if he'd like the alternatives—disease and child-support payments.

When it comes to logistics, remember the Boy Scout motto and be prepared. Keep a condom in your wallet or a discreet pocket of your purse. Do *not* be offended if it turns out he's brought one along on your first date. Guys may *hope* to "get lucky," but they don't necessarily plan on it. (Come to think of it, a lot of us gals are the same way.) He deserves props, not criticism, for being prepared.

Even if you know you're going to be at his place, bring a condom along, and keep your purse where it's accessible. Most guys will be smart enough to keep their stash next to the bed, but you don't want to take the chance of him having to root around under his bathroom sink. At your place, keep a few condoms in your nightstand or a pretty box just for this purpose. You'll know when the moment's right.

SEPTEMBER

Position of the Week: The Placid Embrace

Sir Richard Francis Burton's translations of the *Kama Sutra*, *Ananga Ranga*, and *The Perfumed Garden* give us not only a picture of the sexual mores of ancient cultures, but the Victorian fascination with all things Indian and exotic. In his footnotes to the section in the *Ananga Ranga* that deals with positions, Burton reminds his readers that many of the positions described are "absolutely impossible" for Europeans. The goal of sex for the ancient Hindu, Burton adds, was "to avoid tension of the muscles, which would shorten the period of enjoyment… even in the act of love, he will delay to talk, to caress his wife, to eat, drink, chew Pan-supari, and perhaps smoke a water pipe." In other words, the ancients took snack breaks! Perhaps Burton was reminding his prudish Victorian society that sex was not something to be rushed through guiltily, but savored and enjoyed.

According to the *Ananga Ranga*, The Placid Embrace refers "to a form of congress much in vogue amongst the artful students of the Kamashastra," another ancient sex manual. You can see why it was so popular, because it seems designed to lengthen your period of enjoyment as long as possible. You lie on your back as your man lifts your buttocks while entering you from a kneeling position. He then slips his hands under you to support your back. Twine your legs around his torso, and cross your ankles to pull him closer if you'd like. Reach up and clasp your hands around his neck. While hardly as placid as its name would imply, this position encourages you to express your deep tenderness and passion toward one another.

SEPTEMBER

Two Heads Are Better Than One

Double your pleasure with a double-headed massager. These vibrators feature two vibrating heads placed several inches apart—perfect for stimulating your vaginal and anal regions at the same time. Most come in two speeds, fast and slow, and they pack a wallop. They're not light, either. The Hitachi Magic Twin Head Massager, which looks like a handheld mixer sporting two tennis balls, weighs 2.4 pounds and comes with a fairly steep price tag. At forty watts, it's also one of the strongest massagers on the market. You can get more out of it by experimenting with attachments like the Wonder Wand, a blue vinyl attachment designed for vaginal or clitoral stimulation, or the G-Spotter, which provides G-spot or prostate massage. Or try both attachments at once!

The other type of double-headed massager looks like a curved wand with two small bulbs at the end. The HoMedics Percussion Massager, for example, features two pivoting heads that deliver 3,100 pulses per minute. While you can't buy attachments that allow penetration, the massager itself comes with four attachments designed to vary the intensity of the massage—and even deliver heat!

Don't forget that you can always use your dual-headed massager for the purpose it was intended, namely, giving each other a wonderful, intense massage. Try running the two heads down your partner's back to ease out the knots and get him in the mood!

SEPTEMBER

Cut the Cord: Battery-Operated Vibrators 101

Battery-operated vibrators have gained a loyal following for many reasons, including their low price, versatility, and best of all, portability. With a battery vibe, you're no longer tethered to an electrical cord and power outlet. Take your vibe anywhere: On long drives! On camping trips! On vacation! To parties! Movie theaters! All you need are a couple of C or AA batteries, and you've got portable pleasure.

Battery-powered vibrators come in a wide assortment of colors, shapes, sizes, and styles. Some even come with fun attachments. Remember, however, that it's the vibration, not the size, that delivers the pleasure. Battery vibes deliver gentler vibrations than their electric counterparts, and a toy powered by three C batteries will pack more punch then one that runs on one AA. However, many battery vibes these days offer variable speed control: You simply turn the base to increase or decrease the intensity. Some vibrators even have control panels that let you program the speed and rotation, while other models feature a battery pack that you can hand over to your lover, allowing him to dial up your pleasure.

The downside to battery-operated vibrators is that their low cost sometimes translates into low quality. In general, you get what you pay for, but do some comparison-shopping. And before you plunk down your cash, consider the purpose for which you want your toy: Do you want one that's waterproof? Realistic? Simultaneous clitoral/vaginal or vaginal/anal stimulation? "All of the above" is a fine answer, too. With all the fun models on the market, there's no reason not to fill your toy chest.

SEPTEMBER

Taking Care of Your Toys

It's important to take care of your toys, so they can take care of you for many years to come. Keep them in a cool, dry place, like a dresser or nightstand drawer, wrapped in silk scarves. Take the batteries out when you're not using your vibe: This prevents it from getting left on, which will wear down the batteries (and could be a bummer at an inopportune moment), and ensures that the batteries don't leak. Unplug your coil or wand vibrator so it doesn't overheat.

Inexpensive battery vibrators are often lacking in the quality department, so don't be too surprised if your cheap model conks out when you least expect it. (It doesn't hurt to have an extra toy, and a supply of batteries, on hand.) If your battery vibe does go on the fritz, it might mean some dust has gotten in there. Try blowing on the parts, and make sure that the batteries are inserted correctly.

Say you've had your fun and enjoyed your afterglow, and it's now time to clean up. Clean nonporous vibrators—such as those made from vinyl, hard plastic, or latex—with mild soap and water, but be careful not to immerse your vibe in water unless you're sure it's waterproof. Rinse well and airdry. You can clean silicone, which is completely nonporous, in the same way. With porous toys like rubber or cyberskin, use a condom (clean-up's a snap!) or wash with mild soap and water, rinse, and dry with a clean cloth. Dust cyberskin vibrators with cornstarch—*not* talcum powder, which has been linked to cervical cancer—before storing.

SEPTEMBER

Awakening the Sixth Chakra

Your sixth chakra, also known as the brow chakra, is located between your eyebrows. Also referred to as the "third eye," this energy center governs your powers of intellect: perception, intuition, imagination and visualization. Some believe it even holds sway over our psychic powers. Think of it as the place where your inner light resides—the light that illuminates your inner wisdom, your ability to discern reality from fantasies, and the deepest parts of your being.

Your brow chakra becomes blocked when you close your eyes to the truth. You can reopen it through practices such as yoga, meditation, and visualization. Even if you don't believe in chakras, these activities are proven stress-relievers and help calm overactive minds so that you can hear the messages your "self" is trying to send you over the noise of day-to-day life.

A caring lover can also help you open your third eye. Tantrikas believe that in fact, the third eye opens during orgasms. First, though, practice meditating on the spot between your brows. Sit in a comfortable, sturdy chair or on a couch. You may want to gaze at a candle flame, close your eyes, and then visualize the flame. Roll your eyes back into your head and allow yourself to surrender. Once you feel comfortable with this meditation, focus on your third eye, your eyes rolled back in your head, while your partner pleasures you. Note what happens at the moment of an orgasm, if you have one. Some people report visions, while others see white lights or experience overwhelming spiritual bliss. Enjoy whatever experience you have, and see what it tells you about your inner self.

SEPTEMBER

Lighting Your Internal Fire

In Tantra, *Kundalini* refers to the universal goddess (or Shakti) energy of creation. Tantrikas believe that your Kundalini energy lies coiled at the base of your spine, waiting to be awakened, which is the reason it's often represented by a snake. By stimulating your Kundalini and drawing it up through your body, you can create powerful states of sexual and spiritual ecstasy. There are several ways to begin safely awakening your Kundalini. One is by Kundalini shaking, which helps energy begin moving around the pelvis, preparing you for lovemaking.

Play some fast, rhythmic music that makes you want to dance, such as world beat or Sufi music. Stand with your feet apart about hip width, arms relaxed, and knees soft. Close your eyes. Start shaking your hips and shoulders in time to the music. The faster you shake, the better. Don't worry about how you look—you can always pretend you're a bellydancer. Think about shaking all the tension out of your body. Sing or make noises if that helps you relax your jaw and throat. As you shake, feel the energy building around your abdomen and pelvis. After several minutes, start slowing down. Come to a stop, then sit or lie down to let yourself feel the dynamic energy coursing through your body.

When you're working with Kundalini, easy does it. "I experienced a spontaneous emergence of my Kundalini energy during a meditation exercise," says my friend Clara, a publisher. "My energies were out of control to the degree that I would have spontaneous orgasms in traffic. Someone else I knew even had them while sitting in church. From that point on, I knew why some of those celibate yogis always had smiles on their faces!"

SEPTEMBER

Position of the Week: The Splitting Position

When you start reading many ancient love manuals, you'll see that many of the sexual positions closely resemble each other. It's not really that surprising, because there are only so many positions for intercourse. What's fun is seeing the interesting names and subtle differences writers gave these positions.

Take The Splitting Position of the *Ananga Ranga*. It's fairly simple: You lie on your back as your kneeling partner enters you. Then he lifts both of your legs up and rests them on one shoulder. The position is almost identical to With Legs in the Air, described in *The Perfumed Garden*, which was written hundreds of years earlier in fifteenth-century Tunis. The Sheikh, however, advises his male readers to "raise her legs until the soles of her feet look at the ceiling." And on the other side of the world and a few hundred years earlier, seventh-century physician Li T'ung Hsüan described virtually the same position in his Taoist pillow book *T'ung Hsüan Tzu*. He called it The Dragon Turns.

By keeping your knees and thighs close together, you'll increase the friction on his penis. He'll be able to penetrate you deeply, but you'll get almost no stimulation to your clitoris unless you do it yourself or he reaches between your thighs.

SEPTEMBER

Libra: Tipping the Scales

If your birthday falls between September 23 and October 22, you fall under the astrological sign of Libra, symbolized by the scales. Astrologers consider Librans to be refined, intelligent, warm, and social people who love comfort and luxury, and who weigh decisions carefully (sometimes to the point of indecision). Romantic Librans crave relationships, but often prefer an intellectual connection over deep emotional intimacy or physical passion.

Librans are natural people-pleasers, so if this is your sign, take care that you don't neglect your own sexual needs to accommodate the wishes of your partner. If you do so, you'll end up resenting him—a one-way ticket to anger, depression, and the end of a relationship. Instead, take some time to get to know your own sexual responses and likings. Librans also are very concerned with physical appearance—their own and others'—so you may have to focus on "letting go" during lovemaking. Don't worry about how you look when you're in the throes of passion. You look sexy, and it drives your man wild.

When it comes to sex, your Libra man will respond well to your efforts to create the perfect ambiance for romance. Low lighting, soft music, luxurious bedsheets—your Libran will love anything that sets an elegant mood, and that makes him feel pampered and fawned over. In bed, you'll be rewarded by a caring, generous partner who really wants to please you. Make sure you don't neglect his needs, though—although you may have to work a little bit to help him discover what they are!

SEPTEMBER

Learn about His Family Jewels

In most discussions about sex, the penis gets all the attention. But what about its neighbors, the scrotum and testicles? Most women have no idea what to do with them, so we tend to ignore them entirely. But this is missing a great opportunity to enhance your man's pleasure.

First, understand what you're dealing with. The testicles are glands involved in the production of testosterone and sperm, while the scrotum is the loose sac of skin that contains and protects them. A man's balls can change shape, size, and even location depending on the circumstances. For example, when he's warm, they might hang loose, but when he's cold or aroused, the muscles in his scrotum pull them closer to his body. Don't be alarmed if one testicle hangs lower than the other. This is completely common and completely natural.

As most of us are aware, there's not much a man fears more than being kicked or punched in this region. So approach his equipment with extreme delicacy and a tender, soothing touch—at least at first. Hold them in the palm of one hand, and trace gentle figure eights around them with the other. "Make your tracings random," advises one male friend, "to avoid predictability and focus his attention on what you're doing." Once he knows you intend only the best for his family jewels, he may welcome some vigorous polishing. We'll get to that tomorrow.

BONUS TIP: Think of his testicles as a single entity. Never squeeze them so hard that they separate.

SEPTEMBER

Play Ball!

Now that you've met the testicles, how do you play with them nicely? Say hello by reaching underneath them and lightly stroking the smooth spot on the underside with your middle finger. When you're ready to move on, make a ring with your thumb and index finger at the top of his sac, with his testicles resting in the palm of your hand. Pull gently downward on his scrotum as you stroke his penis or pleasure him with your mouth. Time the downward strokes with the rhythm of your hand or mouth.

This technique will work whether he's on his back with you between his knees, or if you're lying down while he straddles your waist. Use one hand to stroke his erection, and another to fondle his jewels. Or, with your stroking hand, glide from the tip of his penis all the way down to his sac. One friend described some other creative moves: "Hold his penis with the tip pointed at his belly button, and tap his testicles lightly with your finger. Then hold his penis and scrotum with your thumb and forefinger around the base like a loop. Gently pull them forward and move them the left, right, up and down, as though you were moving a joystick. This usually won't get him to climax, but it will result in a bigger orgasm when you do get around to it!"

While some men love to have their testicles fondled, others could care less. Check with your man to ensure that he is enjoying your ball-playing abilities. At the very least, he'll likely be delighted that you're paying attention to this oft-neglected part of his sexual anatomy.

SEPTEMBER

Rev Up Your Fantasy Engine

Are your fantasies feeling tired and lifeless? Do what artists do when they need to "prime the pump:" Open yourself to all possible sources of inspiration. Read erotica, and imagine yourself as one (or all) of the characters. Scan the photo layouts in adult magazines. Check out the *Letters to Penthouse* book series. Thumb through sex advice books. Rent erotic movies. When you see a handsome stranger, make up a daydream involving him.

Got a tried-and-true fantasy? Why not arouse yourself in a new way by writing it down, elaborating, and embellishing as you see fit? (You may end up having to type with one hand.) Learn more about your fantasy style from books like *In the Garden of Desire* by Wendy Maltz and Suzie Boss, or Jack Morin's *The Erotic Mind*.

It pays to keep your erotic imagination humming: Researchers have found that some women, especially ones who are already easily orgasmic, can climax through fantasies or dreams alone. And a study in the *Journal of Sex Research* found that for some people, fantasies make the difference between achieving an orgasm or not. But if you find you don't need fantasies to enjoy sex, that's perfectly okay. Fantasizing isn't a requirement for sexual ecstasy, but it can be a lot of good, clean fun.

SEPTEMBER

Help! There's a Student in the House!

Remember those days when you were a teenager and used to worry about your parents catching you petting on the couch? Now that you've got a teen of your own, you'll realize that you're facing the reverse problem—you have to worry about your teenager catching *you*. It's a safe bet that there's not much a teen would find more horrifying than overhearing his parents in the act. So what do you do when your pubescent kid is staying up late studying for his or her biology midterms, and you don't want to inadvertently give him or her a real-life lesson on human sexuality?

Turn it around to your advantage. Channel the fear of being overheard by your mortified teenager into deliciously long foreplay as you wait for him or her to fall asleep. "Sometimes we'll even start 'foreplay' earlier in the evening, with little secret touches while we're fixing dinner," says my friend Anne. "We can hardly wait to get into bed." Once they're sequestered in their bedroom, the effort of trying to keep quiet gets both of them really hot and bothered, heightening the anticipation and the erotic thrill. "Sometimes my husband even has to put his hand over my mouth!" Anne giggles.

SEPTEMBER

Sex and Chemistry

There are many substances that dull our senses and make it harder for us to achieve orgasms. Alcohol may relax you and your inhibitions, but it also dries up your mucous membranes, decreasing your natural vaginal lubrication. (Marijuana and over-the-counter cold medications can have the same effect.) So if you think you're going to be knocking boots, limit yourself to one or two drinks, if any. Half a glass of red wine is all it takes to raise your testosterone levels, enhancing sex. Another way to help your sex life is to quit smoking. Tobacco constricts blood circulation and may lower your testosterone. Studies have shown that smoking may increase impotence by as much as fifty percent—and can interfere with a woman's ability to achieve an orgasm.

For some people, antidepressants can cause decreased libido, reduced sensation and lubrication, and difficulty achieving orgasms. Extra lubrication can help—as will patience. You may need to stay on antidepressants for a short time to help you get though a bad time; controlling your depression may outweigh the sexual side effects, and your body may adjust to your medication. However, do talk to your doctor. It could be that a different medication will interact differently with your body chemistry.

The other side of the coin is that depression itself can cause a lack of libido, and some studies have shown that depressed people are more likely to engage in unsafe sex. Treating your depression with therapy and medication may allow you to work on the self-esteem issues that are so crucial to a great sex life and fabulous, satisfying orgasms.

SEPTEMBER

Rx for Orgasms?

For the many people who suffer from sexual dysfunction, modern science is providing new options. Medications like Viagra, Levitra, and Cialis work by increasing blood flow to the penis, allowing a man to get and hold an erection *if he is sexually excited.* These drugs are not aphrodisiacs: They won't increase his libido, or give him an instant erection. Nor are they for every man: Men who have cardiovascular disease should not take Viagra, for example. Check with your doctor. And for women? In studies, Viagra has shown some positive results for postmenopausal women, but studies involving younger women have so far shown little or no benefits.

When testosterone levels are low, both men and women may experience low libido. Testosterone patches and gels are prescribed for men, but the FDA hasn't approved their use for women suffering from low libido (what's up with that?). Some companies, however, are conducting experiments, particularly in the use of testosterone in combination with estrogen.

Please talk your doctor if you want to explore any of these medications. Although it's tempting to slap a label like "female sexual dysfunction" on problems like decreased libido or orgasm difficulties, make sure you've explored other options before popping a pill. A prescription is no cure for lack of foreplay or emotional considerations, like not trusting your partner. Don't expect yourself to go from zero to sixty in five seconds without the mental and physical stimulation that you may need to enjoy loving sex and incredible, blissful orgasms.

SEPTEMBER

Position of the Week: The Turning Position

The *Kama Sutra* and other erotic texts occasionally describe positions that seem more like dares than ways to make love. The Turning Position is one of these positions. After starting out in the basic man-on-top position, the man turns around on the woman—without withdrawing his penis—as if he were a giant top. Here's how to try it if you want to go for a perfect ten in a sexual gymnastics competition:

+ First, he enters you in the standard missionary position, supporting himself up on his arms so that his upper body is clear of yours.

+ He then lifts first one leg and then the other over one of your legs.

+ Next, he turns so that he body is perpendicular to yours (you'll be forming a giant human cross).

+ He keeps turning so that his upper body ends up between your legs with one leg on either side of your shoulders.

Here are some ways to cheer him on while he's attempting this tricky maneuver. Caress and stroke his chest, thighs, and finally, his butt (you'll be staring right at it, so you might as well). Keeping your legs slightly parted will help him stay inside you as he's turning. Until he's staring at your feet, don't thrust—this is one time when it's okay to just lie there. Remember, he should turn *slowly* so as not to injure his member. You can see why Vatsyayana advised that this position is "learnt only by practice."

CHAPTER TEN

OCTOBER

"There is something in October that sets the gypsy blood astir."
—*William Bliss Carman,* **A Vagabond Song**

October naturally brings thoughts of Halloween, the most popular fall holiday. This month will lead up to that deliciously wicked evening with all sorts of naughty role-playing and other erotic games. It's a perfect time to overcome your inhibitions. Trick or treat, anyone?

In the Victorian language of flowers, this month's birth flower, the *calendula*, represented joy. Also known as the pot marigold, calendula's yellow and orange blossoms were used by sixteenth-century herbalists in broths and teas to comfort the heart and soothe the spirit. However you decide to use it, let the sight of a calendula flower remind you to let joy into your lovemaking.

October's birthstone is the shimmering *opal*, long treasured for its beauty and protective powers. Giving someone an opal as a gift is symbolic of confidence and faithfulness. So give one to yourself, as a symbol that this month, you're going to be confidently faithful to your heart's desire!

OCTOBER

Harvest Celebration

A remnant of a time when people lived off the land, harvest festivals have been celebrated for thousands of years. In Britain and Australia, people celebrate the Harvest Home festival in late September or early October by decorating churches with fruits and vegetables, and enjoying a harvest supper.

Create your own harvest festival with a sensual banquet just for two. In this banquet, however, there won't be any tables, chairs, or utensils. Instead, serve the food upon your body or his for the other person's dining pleasure! Spread out a towel or blanket on your living room floor (make sure it's one you don't mind getting messy), then get creative with your culinary efforts. Assign different courses to different body parts. Arrange grapes between and around your breasts. Paint your bodies with whipped cream, syrup, yogurt, or ice cream. Drink wine or liqueur from each other's belly button; have him drizzle champagne over your labia. Imagine the potential for vegetables like cucumbers, baby carrots, and zucchini. If things degenerate into a food fight, don't worry about it. Later, you can always take a hot bath together!

OCTOBER

Celebrate Oktoberfest

The two-week beer festival known as Oktoberfest is celebrated annually around this time of year. Oktoberfest festivities have spread throughout the world, but you don't have to travel outside your bedroom to enjoy the pleasures of beer. The following tips, courtesy of my good friend Kyle, work great on a hot Indian summer night—or in front of a roaring fireplace on nippy fall evenings.

Play with the sensations of hot and cold against bare skin by taking an ice-cold bottle of beer and running it over your guy's bare chest. Tease the tip of his nipples with the bottom of the bottle. Cover one nipple with the opening of the bottle, and tip it upwards so it forms a seal. Let the bubbles send shivers down his spine, then remove the bottle and lick the beer off his nipples. "This drives *every* guy crazy," Kyle assures me. Dribble a few drops of beer on his chest, or on either side of his neck, and lick these off, too. Run the bottle's icy cold surface down his abs to his inner thighs, and then up to this testicles and the base of his penis.

You'll win points not only for liking beer (extra bonus points if it's Märzen, the special Oktoberfest beer), but also for being one of the coolest and most creative lovers he's ever had. And of course, a turn about is fair play. Hand the bottle to him, and let him go to work on you.

SAFETY TIP: Do *not* insert anything that could break—like the neck of a bottle—into the vagina or anus.

OCTOBER

Build Your Erotic Library

Looking for ways to spark your libido? Many people find reading erotic literature, either by themselves or with a partner, to be tremendously arousing. And these days, it's easier to find erotic reading material than ever before—which makes the chances of finding something that appeals to you much better. How do you judge whether something's erotic? Simply put, it turns you on. In order to accomplish that, you'll need a clear, honest acceptance of what gets you hot and bothered.

Where do you find erotica? Most chain bookstores carry it, although you may have to scout around (look in the Sexuality section). You can also try alternative and independent bookstores; retail stores like Good Vibrations; and mail-order and online catalogs, like the Venus Book Club, which specializes in sex. Amazon.com's large inventory and customer reviews ensure that you'll find something you'll like.

A good way to start building your erotic library is by checking out the annual erotica anthologies like *Best American Erotica* (Simon & Schuster), *Herotica* (Down There Press), and *Best Women's Erotica* (Cleis Press). These collections feature high-quality writing from a variety of authors, and stories written for almost every sexual orientation and taste. Once you find something you like, you can zero in on your specific preference, whether it's as general as "erotica written by women" or as specific as "bondage erotica." After finding what you like, you'll have another good reason to curl up with a good book on a cold winter's night.

OCTOBER

More Fodder for Your Erotic Reading List

What if you want to venture beyond the annual erotica anthologies? Check out these genres for erotic literature:

+ **Women's erotica:** Erotic fiction by women is striking out towards new frontiers. Expect to see hot stories about women of every shape, age, ethnicity, and sexual preference in collections like *Herotica, Best Women's Erotica, Best Lesbian Erotica,* and *Best Bisexual Women's Erotica.*

+ **Multicultural erotica:** Today's erotica market features voices from a variety of cultural perspectives, with stories and anthologies geared toward African-American, Asian, Latino, and Jewish communities, among others.

+ **Gay erotica:** Erotica and porn featuring gay men are finding a growing number of fans among heterosexual women and lesbians. Why? Because for the most part, it unabashedly depicts graphic sex, and lots of it. Try series like *Best Gay Erotica* or collections such as *Just the Sex.*

+ **Mass-market:** Look for inexpensive, paperback collections or novels featuring highly explicit and delightfully lecherous writing, such as the Black Lace or The Marketplace series. It's not great literature, but that's not why you're buying it, are you?

+ **Literary:** Some of our best writers have produced sexually explicit work: Consider Henry Miller, Anaïs Nin, Anne Rice, and Nicholson Baker.

The list doesn't end there, of course. There's S&M erotica by the truckloads. Science fiction erotica. Supernatural erotica. Gothic erotica. Horror erotica. You name a sexual proclivity, someone's explored it in fiction. So what's on *your* reading list?

OCTOBER

More Moves for High-Intensity Lovemaking

Here are some more tips for increasing the sensations for both of you during intercourse. You know how good it feels when you hold open your labia during oral sex, stretching the skin around the clitoris tight? Try pressing down on the skin at the base of his penis, as you do during oral or manual sex. This keeps the skin of his penis taut, making the friction even stronger as he thrusts.

One male friend of mine strongly advises a woman to squeeze her PC muscles as her man begins to climax. "Sometimes, this can even result in a second orgasm if the squeeze is sufficiently strong," he says. This same friend also recommends pressing on a man's perineum (the point between his scrotum and anus) with gentle, but firm, pressure. If done at the right moment, this move can greatly intensify his orgasm.

Consult *The Perfumed Garden* for other more erotic movements to try during lovemaking. In the Love's Tailor move, your man inserts his member partway and then thrusts quickly and shallowly before burying himself into you up to the hilt, like a tailor plunging his needle into cloth. With The Toothpick in the Vulva move, he thrusts up and down, right and left. "Only a man with a very vigorous member can execute this movement," the author advises. The Sheikh calls The Boxing Up of Love the best of all movements. Your man slides into you deeply, "so closely that his hairs are completely mixed up" with yours, and moves forcibly. Be sure to make good use of your PC muscles!

OCTOBER

Ballplaying in the Major Leagues

Don't forget about your man's testicles and scrotum during oral sex. Drive him wild by licking or blowing over the skin. You can also thrill him by sucking gently on one or both of his testicles.

You may have heard about a technique called "teabagging" on an episode of *Sex in the City*. Basically, this is when you take both of his testicles into your mouth. Use the basic position—thumb and forefinger in a loop around the sac—and pull down until you have a nice little package. (Having him straddle you gets gravity working in your favor.) Cover your teeth with your lips before applying your oral skills. As with any other skill, practice makes perfect.

Even though we've discussed manual and oral techniques for his testicles, don't forget his jewel pouch during lovemaking. If you're on top, you can stroke his testicles whether you're facing towards his head or towards his feet. In the missionary position, reach under your leg or between your bodies. Be sure to keep your movements smooth and gentle, not jerky. Note that for many guys, one of the biggest turn-ons about the rear entry is the lusty sensation of their balls slapping rhythmically against your thighs. Reach through your legs and see if a few strokes to his *cojones* won't heighten the sensation.

OCTOBER

Positions of the Week: Gaping and Encircling Positions

The ancients viewed sex as an art form to be enjoyed by both parties. The *Ananga Ranga*, for example, stresses the importance of foreplay to a woman's pleasure: "These embraces, kisses and sundry manipulations must always be practised according to the taste of husband and wife, and if persisted in… they will excessively excite the passions of the woman, and will soften and loosen her Yoni so as to be ready for carnal connection."

In the Gaping Position, you lift your hips and arch your body to meet his by placing pillows or cushions under your lower back and derriere. Your man then kneels on a pillow himself to raise himself to the right height before entering your "seat of pleasure." The position opens your legs, and thus your genitals, to more stimulation. "This is an admirable form of congress," says the author, "and is greatly enjoyed by both." I'll say!

The Encircling Position is a bit more elaborate. Lie on your back, cross your legs at the calves and raise your knees toward your head. Again, your man kneels in front of you as he slips into your vagina, which will be framed by your legs and feet. "This position is very well fitted for those burning with desire," says Malla, and indeed, you may find the sensation of being pinned down, your vulva and clitoris open to his plundering, highly arousing.

OCTOBER

A Trip to Fantasyland

Your brain is a marvelous storehouse of memories, images, and fantasies that can provide you with an endless source of sexual arousal. In your fantasies, you can make love with whomever you choose, whenever you want, and in any way you desire, with absolutely no repercussions. Your fantasies can be elaborate sexual scripts, or simply images that pass through your mind.

To encourage richer, more enjoyable fantasies, don't limit yourself to "safe" fantasies or censor your fantasies as too outlandish or kinky. People fantasize about all sorts of activities they would never pursue in real life: Sex with people other than their current squeeze (especially celebrities); voyeurism and exhibitionism; forced sex; sex with someone of the same sex; "gang bangs" and group sex; and S&M. All are common fantasy themes.

Don't worry about fantasies that involve taboo or "politically incorrect" activities either. First, there's no indication that fantasizing about something means that you're going to do it. You may fantasize about it *because* it's something you'd never do. Taboos are erotic almost by definition; people are always tantalized by the forbidden. Or maybe your fantasy represents an aspect of your personality that isn't finding expression—an unassertive woman might fantasize about becoming a dominatrix, or a Type A businesswoman might pleasure herself to visions of erotic submission to a cruel "master." Dig deep into the well of your sexual fantasy, and see what it has to teach you, but go easy on yourself. Let your imagination go wild!

OCTOBER

Cut the Cord: Battery-Operated Vibrators 102

When you say "vibrator," what most often comes to mind is the cylindrical variety. Generally, these come in two models—smooth and realistic. "Smoothies" are straight, smooth, and generally made of hard plastic, although you can also find rubber, cyberskin, or silicone versions. Available in a wide variety of colors, smoothies range in size from four to eight inches long, about one-and-a-quarter-inch wide, and usually have a variable speed control at the base (although some have a battery pack attached by a cord that puts the controls within easy reach). Smoothies deliver the strongest vibrations of all of the cylindrical vibrators.

"Realistic" vibrators are what they sound like: Vibrators designed to look and feel like a real penis. Sometimes they even have veins, testicles, and what passes for realistic skin texture. These can be a nice addition to your fantasies, with or without a partner. Remember, however, that no matter how much it looks like a penis, your realistic toy's vibrations probably aren't going to do much inside you unless you add some clitoral stimulation. But you may love the feeling of being penetrated—the vibrations echoing throughout your vagina—while you pleasure yourself with your fingers.

If you like variety, many cylindrical toys come with vinyl sleeves that let you change the look and feel of your vibrator. Their nubs and fringes may not provide much sensation inside you, but if your clitoris is sensitive, they might provide you with some thrilling and arousing sensations.

OCTOBER

When Two Vibrations Are Better Than One

If you want to double your pleasure, consider a dual-action vibrator. Imagine a vibrating shaft that rotates and swivels inside you *and* a small clitoral knob pressing against your love button. Or a little twig that branches off the shaft to tickle your delicate anal opening. Sometimes the main shaft even contains small beads designed to stimulate the sensitive outer third of your vagina. These "twice as nice" vibrators cost a little more, but many people swear by them. Invest in models like the original Rabbit Pearl (cheap imitations have been recalled).

By the way, don't be alarmed if the clitoral vibe on your dual-action toy looks like a tiny bunny with twitching ears or a fetching beaver with a flapping tongue. On one model, the Blue Hawaiian, the snout of a tiny bottle-nosed dolphin will tickle your fancy. In Japan, where these toys were originally launched, it used to be illegal to make sex toys that looked like penises, so manufacturers began coming up with creative alternatives. The tradition continues to this day.

Your dual-action vibe may have a flashing tip, an LED control panel, and a design out of science fiction. If you like novelty *and* the incredible combination of internal and external vibrations, add one of these toys to your shopping list. Just make sure it's not too long, because cute bunny ears won't do much good if they can't reach you where it counts!

OCTOBER

Self-Loving Reason #10: It's the Safest Sex!

One of the many nice things about masturbation is that it's probably the safest sexual activity you can engage in. When you make love to yourself, you obviously don't have to worry about getting pregnant or contracting an uncomfortable and possibly life-threatening disease. You also don't have to worry about whether you've had sex too early in your relationship or whether you're going to call yourself the next day. When it's just you, it's perfectly okay to be easy.

With your partner, masturbation is safe, enjoyable, and stress-free, because it relieves you not only of health worries but also the need to rely on his honesty about his sexual history. Forgot the condoms? Think of the fun you can have without exchanging bodily fluids! You can pleasure each other with your hands or his, dildos, vibrators, and other sex toys. (If you're going to share a vibrator or dildo, remember that a condom can be easily removed and replaced before it goes from one person to the other.) As we discussed on August 6, mutual masturbation can be both erotic and educational, because you get to show each other exactly how you like it, and you get to see how aroused he gets watching you pleasure yourself. So be safe: Masturbate!

OCTOBER

The Magic Bullet

If you want powerful stimulation to your clitoris, vibrating eggs deliver the goods—and the ecstasy. Made of hard plastic or plastic wrapped in vinyl, jelly rubber, or cyberskin, they're slightly smaller than a real egg and attached by a cord to a battery pack that lets you control the intensity of the sensation. Sometimes, they're shaped like—and called—bullets.

By grasping the egg or bullet between your fingers, you can slide it into your vagina and let it nestle inside you. You can even wear it under your clothes! (Everyone will wonder why you look so happy at the next staff meeting.) Or hand the controls over to your man and let him send you to ecstasy while he pleasures your sensitive regions. When you're done, don't pull by the cord; instead, reach inside and pull on the bottom as you bear down. You can also rub a bullet or egg vibe lovingly over your clitoris, or insert it into a hollowed dildo or anal toy made especially for this purpose. Imagine the combinations of a dildo inside you while an egg vibrates against your clitoris. Or thrill your man by cupping an egg in your palm and placing it over his throbbing erection. Nice.

OCTOBER

The Element of Surprise

Don't forget the thrill of unexpected, spontaneous sex to keep your love life from becoming mundane. Even if you can't have actual intercourse, you can surprise each other with carnal treats. Unzip his pants while you're watching television—or, if you're really daring, in the back row of a darkened movie theater when there's no one nearby—and give him some hot oral action. Drop to your knees and tease him with your mouth while he's on the phone with his boss.

Many people fantasize about crawling under the white tablecloth of a fine restaurant to perform oral sex on their partner. If you can't pull this off, which is very likely, slip under your dining room table during a romantic candlelight meal at home, or just use your toes or fingers to tease him under the tablecloth. You may find that *you're* dessert.

Waking up to your lover's mouth on you can be deliciously naughty, too. A thirtysomething photographer I know says, "One of the hottest things my wife has ever done to me is bringing me awake with her mouth and then mounting me." Your man may think he's dreaming if you try this, but just think of his excitement when he realizes that he's awake!

OCTOBER

Position of the Week: The Second Posture

It's certainly no secret that some men are as self-conscious about their members as some women are about their thighs. Unscrupulous vendors play off this fear by peddling a variety of products that claim to be able to enlarge or extend shorter penises. It may or may not comfort you that the penis enlargement industry has been going strong for thousands of years. As far back as the sixteenth-century A.D. (and surely even longer), *The Perfumed Garden* devoted an entire chapter to "prescriptions for increasing the dimensions of small members and making them splendid." Some of the solutions Sheikh Nefzawi recommends (poultice of leech, anyone?) are not for the faint of heart.

However, elsewhere the Sheikh recommends very practical positions for making intercourse enjoyable for underendowed men. Whether you would care for them is up for debate. In the Second Posture, you draw your legs back as far over your head as you can—similar to the "plow position" in yoga. By grasping your ankles, you raise your vagina so that your lover can enter you more easily without slipping out. As this position may be hard on your neck and shoulders, you probably won't want to keep it for long. But you'll have fun trying!

OCTOBER

Where's the Remote?

Look, hon, no hands! That's the joy of a remote-controlled vibrator. These toys feature adjustable leg and waist straps that hold a vibrator into place over your clitoris. Microchip technology has helped replace the bulky vibes of old with slim, discreet varieties, like the Remote Butterfly. They still may not be quiet enough to wear in a museum, but imagine the fun at home or at a noisy party.

Unfortunately, one of the downsides to these models is that the elastic straps can be downright confusing or may not hold the vibrator tightly in place, or the vibrator itself may not deliver the stimulation you need. If you have to press down on it, it defeats the hands-free purpose! Consider a panty or thong that comes with a vibrator built into a small pouch. These tend to hold the vibrator more firmly over your clitoris.

You can incorporate "hands-free" vibrators easily into your love-making with a partner. Give the remote to your man so that he can bring you to the point of orgasm again and again, or wear it during intercourse, since the vibrator will usually only cover your clitoris. If yours is a thong, simply move the strap to one side!

HISTORICAL NOTE: Today is the birthday of Dr. Maria Stopes (1880-1958), the English pioneer of the birth control movement who founded the first birth control clinic in England with her husband, Humphrey Verdon Roe.

OCTOBER

Toys for Your Breasts

Are you one of those women who thrills to nipple stimulation? Do you like to have your nipples stroked, teased, or even pinched? Then you may really get a charge out of toys like nipple clamps, which deliver intense stimulation for both men and women. Look for clamps with padded vinyl tips. Tweezer clips work well for women because they're expandable to accommodate different nipple sizes; the broad, flat pincers of alligator clips might be more suitable for men. There are vibrating nipple clamps for those who really want a buzz, and even suction toys that come with a hand pump and a battery vibrator. Many nipple clamps are attached to each other with a length of chain, which gives a nice, kinky look. Tug on the chain gently for extra sensations.

Wait until you're aroused before applying your nipple clamps. That way, the pinching will feel titillating rather than painful. Go slow when experimenting for the first time, so you can learn what feels good. You may want to place the clamp behind the tip rather than directly on it. This will be more comfortable, and there will be less likelihood of the clamp falling off. If your toys have a strong bite, try clasping them around your areola first. Release the clamp slowly: you may feel a very strong sensation as the blood flows back. For some people, removing the clamp is as much fun as putting it on!

SAFETY TIP: If you have breast implants or cystic breasts, be careful about playing with nipple clamps. Don't leave them on for more than twenty minutes.

HISTORICAL NOTE: Oscar Wilde (1854-1900), the Irish author of *The Importance of Being Earnest*, was born on this day. Wilde served two years of hard labor in prison after his 1895 conviction for homosexual offenses.

OCTOBER

Ring Around the Love Rod

If you and your man are into long lovemaking sessions, a cock ring may be just the toy for you. Made of either metal, rubber, or leather, cock rings fit around the base of his penis and scrotum and keep the blood from flowing out. This makes his erection firmer, more sensitive, and longer lasting, enhancing intercourse for both of you.

Rubber or latex rings are inexpensive and flexible—and some have little nubs to give you clitoral stimulation (supposedly)—but they're also porous and thus not for sharing. Steel rings can be sterilized, but could be difficult to remove in a pinch. Leather rings, which fasten with snaps or Velcro, are adjustable, easy to remove, and look pretty darn hot. However, they're not the easiest to clean, which is a polite way of saying that they can get a little skanky.

Here's how to help your man put on a cock ring. Start before he's hard (once he's erect, the game's over, unless you've got an adjustable leather model) by tucking one testicle through the ring at a time, and then his penis. He can also wear his ring just around the base of his penis if he wants. In terms of safety, make sure the ring isn't attached too tightly, and use one you can adjust or remove easily. No matter how much fun you're having, don't leave it on for more than twenty minutes, and don't let him fall asleep wearing it.

OCTOBER

Ring! Vibrations for Both of You

Intrigued by yesterday's discussion? Want to take your cock ring play to the next level? Well, technology has come to your rescue with a variety of vibrating rings designed for your pleasure as well as his. Most of these feature a tiny bullet vibrator at one end, usually attached to a battery pack by a cord. There are several varieties, including rings with sleeves into which you can insert your own bullet or egg vibe. Use a cordless model for hands-free play! Some even come with a vibrating anal attachment attached to the same battery pack by a separate cord.

How do you get the most from your vibrating ring? Place it around the base of his penis with the bullet on the bottom to give his family jewels the benefit of the vibrations. To stimulate your love button during lovemaking, rotate it so that the vibrator is on top. If yours has a battery pack, either of you can take control of the intensity of the vibrations.

As with many sex toys, creative manufacturers have come up with several variations that give some vibrating cock rings their own distinct personality. One manufacturer offers a Bunny Ring Vibe, a jelly rubber ring shaped like a rabbit that features a mini-vibrator in the bunny's head and ears that twitch over your clitoris. At Good Vibrations, the best-selling Neptune Ring Vibe boasts a tiny vibrating dolphin—perfect for your Halloween mermaid costume!

OCTOBER

Awakening the Seventh Chakra

Located at the top of your head, your seventh or crown chakra is the energy center that governs your spiritual consciousness and your relationship with your higher self. Awakening your crown chakra is said to allow you to experience the Divine and your connection to the universe. During lovemaking, an awakened crown chakra can allow you to experience tremendous levels of bliss and connection with your partner.

To awaken the crown chakra, explore different forms of meditation and energy work. Here's a simple exercise that will help you raise the energy throughout your body and may help you experience more blissful orgasms. Sit cross-legged or in another comfortable position. Place your hands on your thighs or clasp them in light fists. Inhale gently, filling your lungs with air. Tighten your PC and anal muscles, and let your eyes roll back slightly. If you want, you can tuck your head slightly and pull in your lower belly. Imagine a stream of white energy—like a tiny flame—rising up your spine to the top of your head with each inhalation. Don't force anything. As you exhale, allow an "Ah" to escape your throat to release any energy caught there.

As you become more comfortable with this technique, visualize the light shooting out the top of your head like a fountain as you inhale. You can do this as you exhale as well. If you like, imagine the feeling of an orgasm! Don't be surprised if you feel like you're flying. To ground yourself, imagine the light raining love down over your body as you exhale, showering every part of your body with bliss. Enjoy your cosmic afterglow!

OCTOBER

Role-Playing Game: Goddess and Devotee

As we approach Halloween, let's get into the spirit with a little role-playing. Whether you're in costume or not, assuming a temporary role with your lover can revive the fun, spontaneity, and playfulness of your early relationship. The following Tantric role-playing game is especially nice if you tend to fall into the nurturing role. Tonight, you'll be nurtured and even worshipped!

In this game, you assume the role of Goddess, while your man is your obedient, eager-to-serve devotee. His role is to provide you with sensual and sexual pleasure, and he must do anything you ask of him. He must also ask your permission before doing anything, and you're free to say yes or no without explanation. Your only job is to focus on your needs. Don't worry about reciprocating. You can switch roles another night.

Take some time to set the scene. Light candles in your bedroom, or book a special hotel room. You might start with a hot bath, asking him to wash your body and hair and anoint your body with fragrant lotions and oils. Then move to the bedroom, where you can take things as slowly or as fast as you want. You set the pace! A nice way to start is to sit across from each other and allow him to offer you some words of praise. While he's speaking, all you need to do is smile, send him thoughts of unconditional love, and allow yourself to get in touch with your divine nature. Imagine yourself as a beneficent Hindu or Buddhist goddess, clad in silk and jewels. When he's done, offer him a few words of blessing, and then let him know how he can serve you for the night.

HISTORICAL NOTE: Today is the birthday of Arthur Rimbaud (1865-91), the French symbolist poet whose tempestuous affair with the poet Paul Verlaine was portrayed in the 1995 movie *Total Eclipse*, with Leonardo DiCaprio playing the role of Rimbaud.

OCTOBER

Position of the Week: The Third Posture

Where the *Kama Sutra* and the *Ananga Ranga*, with their poetic descriptions of intertwined couples, treat women as an equal partner in the proceedings, *The Perfumed Garden* of Sheikh Nefzawi is bawdy and humorous, and almost seems to treat women as objects. Discovered by French army officers in North Africa, *The Perfumed Garden* first surfaced as *Le Jardin Parfumé* in France, where the charismatic Captain Richard Francis Burton found it and set about translating it.

Burton didn't shy from giving the work his own unique editorial stamp. "One need only glance at the book to be convinced that its author was animated by the most praiseworthy intentions," Burton writes in the introduction, adding, "What can be more important, in fact, than the study of the principles upon which rest the happiness of man and woman, by reason of their mutual relations?" Burton may have been the first advocate for sex education!

One *Perfumed Garden* position worthy of study is the Third Posture. Similar to the Yawning Position of the *Kama Sutra*, you lie on your back as your man kneels between your legs. With his help if necessary, put one leg on his shoulder and tuck the other under his arm. Because it allows such deep penetration, wait until you're fully aroused before attempting this position. During high levels of sexual arousal, your uterus moves higher and your inner vagina near your cervix balloons in a process called "tenting," which makes deep penetration and thrusting easier and more pleasurable. No wonder *The Perfumed Garden* devotes so much time to foreplay!

OCTOBER

Pleasures of the Orient

According to legend, women in ancient China and Japan inserted *ben wa* balls—egg-shaped hollow balls carved from ivory—into their vaginas, then rocked back and forth until they climaxed from the sensation! Modern ben wa balls are usually two gold-plated balls about three-quarters of an inch in diameter, but they can also be made of silver, plastic, Lucite, or steel. Often they arrive in pretty packages or boxes, making them a perfect sensual gift.

Ben wa balls are easy to use: You simply slip them into your vagina (not your bottom, where they could get lost) and hold them in place while you fool around or go about your daily business. Bear down with your PC muscles to pop them out. Some women hold them lower in their vagina; others try to tuck them behind their G-spot. Note that you probably won't feel them "rolling" around, as your vaginal walls form a snug sleeve that will hold them in place. The sensation will be much more subtle. However, you can "activate" them by using a vibrator, and some women (and men) enjoy the sensations they produce during intercourse.

For stronger sensations, try duotone balls. These are hollow balls about one-and-one-half inches in diameter that are connected by a nylon leash. The balls contain smaller ball bearings. You can find duotone balls in jelly rubber, plastic, or silicone. Some strands have up to four balls. There are even vibrating versions! Slip them into your waiting love canal, tug on the cord, and enjoy the sensations produced by the smaller balls rolling around inside the larger ones. Tease yourself by pulling them out one by one, until you can't stand it any longer!

OCTOBER

Scorpio: The Lure of the Scorpion

If you or your man were born between October 23 and November 21, you fall under the sign of Scorpio, symbolized by a scorpion. Known as the most extreme zodiac sign, Scorpios are thought to be highly passionate, intuitive, and sensitive. If you find yourself mesmerized by someone's intense gaze, chances are that he or she is a Scorpio. A relationship with a Scorpio won't lack for passion, and you can expect to explore the heights and depths of sexual ardor. A Scorpio man is the perfect person with whom to explore your dark side; if you're a Scorpio yourself, you've probably already done some adventuring—or at least fantasized about it!

If you're involved with a Scorpio, seize this opportunity to take a walk on the wild side. Delve into the arousing potential of erotic videos, literature, role-playing, Tantric sex, and Eastern love manuals. If you're a Scorpio yourself, probe into your own fantasies. As we discuss tomorrow, there are lots of safe, fun ways to explore practices like BDSM (bondage and discipline, domination and submission, and sadomasochism) that don't require you to buy weird leather outfits or scary hardware. Harness the Scorpio passion to recharge your batteries and rediscover the sexual power of the unpredictable and the unknown.

OCTOBER

Kink: It's in the Eye of the Beholder

What makes sex so hot in the early part of a relationship? For the most part, it's because you're discovering the unknown, and that's tremendously exciting. But as a relationship goes on, predictability can set in, and that's the death of eroticism. How do you re-light the spark? You push back the boundaries, and bring back the unex-

pected. There's a way to do this, safely—and make some fantasies come true in the bargain.

Forget your preconceptions about BDSM (bondage and discipline, dominance and submission, and sadomasochism). You don't have to own leather, join a weird club, or think of yourself as deviant. You just have to be willing to explore new sensations and indulge in a little make-believe. And because this kind of sex play requires communication, trust and love, it's perfect for—and most satisfyingly practiced by—those in long-term, secure relationships.

So you're ready to start walking on the wild side. Where do you start? An ideal beginning is consulting books like *The Big Bang: Nerve's Guide to the Sexual Universe* or *The Good Vibrations Guide to Sex,* both of which have excellent guides to S&M play. Then, define your desires. Your sexual fantasies can be a treasure trove of ideas. What elements of your fantasies turn you on the most? Be specific. Some people find it useful to make lists: one list of erotic activities you've tried and liked, and another list of those you'd like to try, and those you'd never do in a million years. These lists give you a road map to the dark side of your erotic psyche, so don't censor yourself. Now, with a loving partner, you're ready to venture forward.

OCTOBER

Power Plays

BDSM takes the subtle power shifts in any human interaction and emphasizes them.(These shifts are there, no matter how much we'd like to deny it.) You can be as bad or as weak as you want, and for once, it's *okay*. In typical BDSM play, the "top" or dominant partner assumes total control, while the "bottom" or submissive partner gives it up in prenegotiated "scenes." A scene can be as simple or as elaborate as your comfort zone allows, but should always be consensual. Maybe the top ties up the bottom and won't let him climax without her permission. Maybe the bottom has been a naughty schoolgirl and deserves a spanking. Maybe the top just wants a two-hour foot rub. It's up to you!

Being the bottom frees you to give yourself completely to another person. You get to be swept away by feeling, and freed from responsibility for your lustful actions. (See March 30 for more.) Being the top, on the other hand, lets you release your inner control freak. You can give free rein to your selfishness, cruelty, and lust for power—typically unattractive qualities in everyday life—all in the context of your partner's pleasure. Everybody wins!

For a fun encounter, communication is key. The more specific you are, the less chance of misunderstanding and disappointment. Don't think of it as lessening the spontaneity—think of it of taking care of the details so you can lose yourself in the moment. Send each other lewd, detailed emails. Scour erotic books and movies together for ideas. Comprise lists of dos and don'ts. Let your planning build your anticipation, because remember: Anticipation is the key to erotic excitement—kinky or not—and excitement is what BDSM is all about.

OCTOBER

Bondage for Beginners

You don't have to truss your partner up like a mummy or invest in scary hardware to enjoy a little loving bondage. Restraints are an easy and fun way to add a little spice to your erotic games. If you have trouble reaching an orgasm, being restrained may free you from pressuring yourself or worrying that you're taking too long.

Restraint materials run the gamut. The safest is probably soft, shiny nylon rope. It's attractive, versatile, easy to clean, and easy to loosen. Clothesline is another inexpensive option, as is PVC or "bondage tape." Silk scarves and stockings are pretty, but they may get too tight and be hard to untie—you'd hate to have to cut up your favorite Hermès scarf. Avoid thin ropes, thread, twine, phone and electrical cord, chain, leather thongs, and yes, handcuffs. In fact, consider investing in restraints made especially for bondage purposes, as they're more comfortable and safer than homemade versions. You might also consult a book like *Jay Wiseman's Erotic Bondage Handbook* for the lowdown on techniques.

Remember: Safety first. Think *sensual bondage*—firm but comfortable. Never tie anyone in a way that cuts off circulation. Leave at least one finger's width diameter between the bond and a wrist or ankle, and keep a pair of blunt-tipped scissors nearby. If someone's limb falls asleep or starts feeling numb, they should speak up, and you should untie them. (Check bound body parts for cooling or numbness every ten to fifteen minutes.) No one should be tied up for more than half an hour or left alone—although you can *pretend* to leave your blindfolded partner and keep an eye on him from afar.

You may not even need to use physical restraints at all. You could simply tell your man "Don't you dare move an inch!" and go to town on him.

OCTOBER

Please, Sir, May I Have a Spanking?

Have you been a very, very bad girl? Maybe you deserve a spanking! Whether it's a quick slap on the butt during intercourse or a carefully administered session during roleplay, many people get a rush from a good slap on the butt. If you're on the receiving end, you may get off on the sensations reverberating throughout your derriere and nether regions. If you're the spanker, you get the excitement of doing something slightly taboo.

Here's a way to get started. The person receiving the spanking (say that's you) decides how many spanks to receive as her "punishment." You then lie over the edge of a couch, on the bed, or over the giver's knee, cheeks exposed. It might be hot for your man to ask you something like, "Are you ready to receive your spanking?" If you are, you answer "Yes, Master," or however you've decided to address him. He then gives you a nice, firm whack on the fleshy part of your behind. Not too hard, not too soft—just enough so it leaves a slight red mark. (When, on another night, it's his turn, you should also aim for his fleshy cheeks, taking extreme care to avoid his testicles.) If it's appropriate for the scene, you can count the spanks out loud and thank him.

As he gives you the negotiated number of spanks, he can increase the intensity, mix it up, or alternate with caressing. How does he know if it's too much? Use your "safe word," an agreed-upon phrase that can't be confused with the expected "Oh please, no more!" of role-playing (see March 29). When he's done, he should caress and soothe your burning buttocks tenderly, or do whatever else you need. Maybe you need to be held, or maybe you'll be so aroused you'll be ready for him to take you then and there!

OCTOBER

Position of the Week: The Seventh Posture

Brilliant, handsome, and magnetic, Captain Sir Richard Francis Burton (1821-1890), the famous explorer who translated the *Kama Sutra*, the *Ananga Ranga,* and *The Perfumed Garden,* lived a life that seems tailormade for Hollywood. He scandalized Victorian society with his publication of ancient erotic texts, but he also challenged Victorian thinking by declaring that women should enjoy sex as much as men.

Of course, your enjoyment of the Seventh Posture from *The Perfumed Garden* may depend on whether you're an advanced yoga students or into Halloween fantasies involving acrobats. To start, you lie on your side and lift one leg to his shoulder—with some help from him—as he straddles your bottom thigh, sitting on his heels, and enters you. As the text implies, your ability to move will be limited; the author advises your man to "make her move by drawing her towards your chest by means of your hands, with which you hold her embraced." Obviously, you may need to roll over slightly onto your back to accomplish this move. It's a nice cross between missionary and side-by-side positions, because it gives you the ability to watch the arousal—or in the case of this position, amusement—playing across each other's features.

OCTOBER

Turn Yourself into a Work of Art

There is an artist inside each one of us, but all too often, our budding creativity was stifled at an early age by someone—a teacher, a parent, a sibling—mocking our fledgling artistic efforts. It's never too late to rediscover our inner artist, and what better way than by using our lover's body as a living canvas! Body painting is a wonderful form of expression that is easy, fun, and much less permanent than a tattoo.

To get started, decide who and what you want to be. Wonder Woman? A leopard? An exotic African parrot? A naughty demon? Get ideas from Web sites like Body Paint Magazine (www. bodypainting.com) or Alteredbody.com (www.alteredbody.com). Then head to your nearest theatrical supply store and look for brands like Mehron. Around Halloween, many costume shops offer body paints as well. Water-based makeup comes off fairly easily in the shower; grease-based takes some scrubbing with baby oil or cold cream. If you plan to get busy with your man, however, make sure you're on sheets you don't mind messing up.

If you don't want to be so elaborate, you can find edible body paints in many stores. Imagine the fun you and your man will have tracing intricate patterns across each other's bodies. With these paints, cleanup is the best part. Just apply your tongue and lick!

OCTOBER

Get into Your Role

Role-playing gives your erotic imagination and creativity free rein, and allows you to bring your hottest fantasies to life. And what could be more fun than enacting an erotic scenario with your man? Perhaps he's the stern professor of sexuality who must instruct his recalcitrant student (you). Or maybe he's the famous porn star demonstrating his technique to the hotshot reporter (you again). Likewise, you might be the pampered rich wife and he's the cabana boy, or you're the Wild West madam and he's the randy cowboy. Maybe he's the four-star general and you're the green recruit! You can even be daring and play your roles in public: biker-barfly, yuppie-Junior Leaguer, whatever. Choose your roles for the effect you want: devotion, subservience, humiliation, punishment. Don't worry about political correctness. This is your chance to play at being an innocent virgin ravished by pirates. Go nuts.

Don't skimp on setting the scene, either. That's part of the fun. Turn your bedroom into a Gothic bedchamber with dripping candles, or a Turkish harem with pillows and silk rugs. If your home reminds you too much of your normal everyday life, book a hotel room. It doesn't have to be expensive: A cheap motel room could be just what your trucker-waitress fantasy needs. Dress the part, too.

During your game, stay in character. Changing your mind halfway through will totally deflate the moment. Throw yourself into your role. You may not win an Oscar, but chances are you'll get a much more exciting erotic reward.

OCTOBER

Trick or Treat!

There's a reason kids like Halloween so much—it's a great excuse to play dress-up! In San Francisco, the yearly Exotic Erotic Ball in October attracts nearly 15,000 revelers who jump at the chance to costume themselves in outrageous, provocative costumes. Dressing sexy can get you in the mood for role-playing, S&M games, and hot sex. If you normally dress like something out of the J.Crew catalog, imagine surprising your man by showing up as a streetwalker.

Dressing up can help you get in the mood for sensual play. If you're going for kinky, look for clothes that emphasize your curves, such as dresses and corsets of tight leather, latex, PVC, or rubber. In some circles, this is known as fetish clothing, but thanks to MTV, it's pretty much entered the mainstream.

Fake fur also adds a touch of decadence. And don't forget props like long gloves, special lingerie, and outrageous high-heeled stilettos. Some people even get turned on by uniforms. Be a policewoman, stern teacher, or sexy nurse. Pretend to be an innocent schoolgirl. Dress up like a maid, dominatrix, slutty sorority girl, UPS delivery woman—wherever your fantasies take you. Then get ready to ring his bell. This Halloween, you'll be getting some very nice (and erotic) treats.

CHAPTER ELEVEN

NOVEMBER

"How well I know what I mean to do / When the long
dark autumn-evenings come."
—Robert Browning (1812-1889), British poet,
Men and Women, *"By the Fire-Side"*

You'll find lots for which to be thankful for this November. As fall brings hints of the first chill and trees prepare to shed their fiery cloaks of red and gold, the following sensual tips will guide you on an erotic pilgrimage of your own, designed to stoke your inner fires and nourish your most secret self in preparation for winter. During these long, dark autumn evenings, we'll give thanks to the gods by celebrating with that most divine gift, the orgasm. This month features a special focus on longer, more heavenly climaxes for both you and your man.

This month's birth flower is the *chrysanthemum*. The Victorians gave each other white chrysanthemums to symbolize truth, and red chrysanthemums to say "I love you." Fill a vase with red and white chrysanthemums as a reminder to be truthful to yourself and your beloved about your sensual needs.

The beautiful *yellow topaz* is this month's birthstone. Legend has it that wearing topaz is said to enhance the ability to give and receive love, resulting in deeper and better relationships.

NOVEMBER

Get Connected

When it comes to sex, all the tips and techniques in the world aren't a substitute for emotional connectedness, the not-so-secret ingredient that makes sex so sweet. When you feel close to your partner, the sex can't help but be great. Nanette, a thirty-two-year-old accessory designer, sums up the sexual energy created when two lovers connect on a deep level:

"During long conversations, my boyfriend and I touch each other's hair, lie on each other's lap, or just sit close to each other. The eye contact and touching, even though it's not sexual, makes both of us feel loved and appreciated, and the lovemaking that always follows is so much more extraordinary. When we kiss, I can feel his desire on my lips. A shock of energy fills my whole being, creating an orgasmic feeling throughout my body that lasts the entire time we're making love. The whole experience feels very sacred, like something only the two of us could achieve together."

It's not just women who need this emotional connection. Men need it, too. We connect with someone on an intimate level when we're able to be ourselves with him or her. During those open, honest conversations, we can be our most authentic selves. So next time you find yourself concentrating on the mechanics of whether you're "doing it right," try connecting with him at an emotional level. Remember all the things you love about him. Go with the flow. Let your actions, and your orgasms, flow from your heart—not your head.

NOVEMBER

Timing Is Everything

The time of day—and even the time of month—can have a significant effect on your orgasms. Your testosterone levels are highest in the morning, heightening your chances for a great orgasm, so set your alarm half an hour early for some early-morning nooky. Or have a nooner. Some studies indicate that your man's testosterone levels, which ebb and flow in twenty-four-hour cycles, peak around mid-day. Whatever you do, don't always wait for bedtime to get busy. It's evening or nighttime when you're most likely to be tired or stuffed from a big dinner, and thus less likely to achieve an orgasm. Speaking of meals, here's another reason for eating light: Having a rich, heavy meal right before sex can make it harder to climax.

Pay attention to your body's workings, too. Thanks to high levels of estrogen, many women report feeling more randy mid-cycle, right before they ovulate. Others feel especially lustful right before their periods, when progesterone drops. Keep going after your period starts: Orgasms help relieve menstrual cramps and backache.

Orgasms aren't always about timing, either: Sometimes they're about time well spent. Don't make a habit of neglecting the kissing and fondling that precedes sex. Research has found that more than ninety percent of women are able to climax after twenty minutes or more of foreplay. But don't worry if you're occasionally pressed for time, because other studies have found that women can achieve orgasms in less than ten minutes with a partner. Sometimes, all it takes to fire up your sex life is a few exciting moments.

NOVEMBER

Fun Orgasm Facts

Here are some quick factoids about the Big O that will keep you lighthearted about your pleasure potential and give you the perfect ice-breakers for cocktail-party chitchat:

+ **Practice makes perfect:** Orgasms aren't instinctual. We discover them by accident and learn how to have them by practice.

+ **Your guy wants to lend a hand:** The Janus Report on Sexual Behavior found that more than half the men surveyed said that their woman's orgasm was more important than their own.

+ **By the numbers:** During an orgasm, women have anywhere from three to fifteen orgasmic contractions. Men have three to four. Both sexes experience these contractions at intervals of eight-tenths of a second. But who's counting?

+ **Built for pleasure:** Women have as much, if not more, erectile tissue than men. It's located throughout our clitoral network, in our clitoris and our clitoral glans, shaft, and bulbs.

+ **Built for stamina:** Most orgasms last for a few seconds of otherworldly bliss, but a woman's orgasm can last up to twenty-eight seconds.

+ **Longest recorded orgasm:** Forty-three seconds with twenty-five consecutive contractions. Lucky!

+ **Every orgasm is different:** Although the experience of an orgasm is subjective, not every orgasm is mind-blowing. Depending on a variety of factors, your experience may range from "That was nice" to momentarily losing consciousness (rare, but it does occur). Know that your orgasms may vary from day to day, so relax. There's no need to go for the gold every time!

NOVEMBER

Position of the Week: The Eighth Posture

When it comes to sex, it seems that there's very little new under the sun. The ancients pilfered freely from each other when composing their famous sex manuals (you'll see similar positions described in the *Kama Sutra*, the *Ananga Ranga,* and *The Perfumed Garden)*. Even Sir Richard Francis Burton, the nineteenth-century translator of these three works, acknowledged that Sheikh Nefzawi borrowed from Arabian and Indian writers in *The Perfumed Garden*, but comments that "it would be ingratitude not to acknowledge the benefit which his books have conferred upon people who were still in their infancy in the art of love." Clearly, the visionary Burton saw that it was all for the greater good.

One *Perfumed Garden* position that echoes early works is The Eighth Posture, which seems very similar to The Encircling Position of the *Ananga Ranga* (see October 7). Cross your legs, your ankles under your calves, and lie back, letting your thighs fall open. Your man kneels astride you "like a cavalier on horseback" and enters you, his hands free to shower you with loving caresses. If he leans forward, he may even be able to stimulate your clitoris with the base of his penis. By changing the position of your hips, this position helps you vary the angle and depth of penetration. Want even deeper penetration or G-spot stimulation? Pull your crossed legs back toward your chest before he enters you, as in the Encircling Position.

NOVEMBER

I'll Have Mine Blended

Did you know that, thanks to the different nerves that surround your pelvic floor muscles, you actually can have several kinds of orgasms? The first kind, experienced by more than seventy percent of women, is a clitoral orgasm. When you massage your clitoris with fingers or a vibrator (or his lusty mouth), you stimulate the pudendal nerve, producing a sharp twinge of arousal. When you have an orgasm, you'll feel the spasms in your genitals.

The second common type is the internal, or vaginal orgasm, which happens when his penis penetrates you deeply against your inner vaginal wall and cervix, stimulating your pelvic and hypogastric (deep vaginal) nerves. The resulting orgasm is often described as warm and "melting." You can achieve it during lovemaking with you on top or him entering you from behind.

Blended orgasms are the best of both worlds. Stimulating both areas at once, or one after another, can result in amazingly intense climaxes. Start by massaging your clitoris, then switching to vaginal penetration, and bring yourself to the brink at least three times before stimulating both areas at once and allowing yourself to climax. Try stimulating your clitoris, vagina, and anus at once for a triple-decker climax.

By the way, despite what Freud claimed, no orgasm is "better" than another. Again, most women need clitoral stimulation to climax.

NOVEMBER

Hands-Free Ecstasy

Believe it or not, it is possible to think your way to an orgasm. Spontaneous orgasms (also called extragenital orgasms) occur when you climax without even touching yourself. Studies have found that more than sixty percent—maybe even one hundred percent—of easily orgasmic women are able to think themselves off through fantasies; these mental orgasms had the same physical symptoms as clitoral or G-spot climaxes. Sexy thoughts can rev up your brain's pleasure center and send you into a high state of arousal. Try watching a sexy movie, reading erotica, or replaying erotic images or memories in your mind until you're over the edge (contracting your PC muscle may help). Some people can achieve "energy orgasms" through breathwork or Tantric techniques.

You can also encourage erotic dreaming. Most people do have sexual dreams from time to time, and up to twenty percent of women actually have experienced sleep orgasms. To encourage this, fill your mind with sensual thoughts and images right before you fall asleep. You might check out books on lucid dreaming like *Creative Dreaming* by Patricia Garfield, which gives practical suggestions for controlling your dreams. In our book *Red Hot Tantra,* my co-author David Ramsdale also discusses erotic lucid dreaming in some depth.

Erotic dreaming can be tons of fun. Just think: In your dreams, you can have all sorts of sexual experiences you would never have in your waking life!

NOVEMBER

Baby, It's You!

Desire ebbs and flows, but there is one time of your life when sex may take a backburner, and that's after childbirth. Go easy on yourself. You've just been through a grueling ordeal. Your body needs a little time to recover, especially if you've had a cesarean birth or any complications from vaginal delivery, perineal tearing, or stitches from an episiotomy. Hormones are working against you. Your estrogen and progesterone levels have dropped dramatically, while prolactin—the hormone that produces breast milk—is not only a natural tranquilizer but reduces vaginal lubrication and makes your genitals less sensitive. And on top of that, you'll be exhausted!

All's not gloom and doom, however. Most couples resume having intercourse within seven weeks or even less. There are certainly other sexual activities in which you can engage, and having to do "everything but," like when you were teenagers, could actually be a turn-on for both of you. Whether you're having manual, oral, or vaginal sex, make sure you're relaxed, and use plenty of lube. A sense of humor will be critical. Ever heard of breast "letdown"? You will. Keep some towels on hand.

Just because your libido's in hiding, you don't have to neglect nonsexual forms of touch—good advice even if you're not dealing with postpartum issues. Hug, kiss, and fondle your partner whenever you have the chance. Exchange foot rubs. Know that eventually your sex life will get back to normal—even if life itself will never be the same again.

NOVEMBER

Good Things Come in Twos, and Threes, and …

In theory, every woman has the ability to experience multiple orgasms—one or more orgasms separated by a few seconds or minutes with no fading of arousal. The reason that women are more likely to experience multiple "Os" has to do with genital blood flow. During a man's orgasm, blood quickly flows out of the penis through a concentrated network of veins. That's why, after they ejaculate, men need a "refractory period" during which they can't have another erection. With women, blood flows in and out more easily—in other words, your genitals stay engorged and ready for action.

Please don't make multiple orgasms another sexual goal and beat yourself up if you can't achieve them. Sex should be pleasure-oriented, *not* goal-oriented. But if you'd like to experiment with it, here's how: After your first orgasm, keep stimulating yourself. Since your clitoris may be too sensitive for direct stimulation, try moving to the surrounding area. For example, caress your inner lips with your vibrator, if you're using one, or rest it on the back of your hand while you continue to touch yourself. Breathe deeply—pant, if you must—and rock your hips. You may feel overstimulated momentarily, but that overstimulation may transform itself into unbelievable pleasure, and another earthshattering orgasm.

NOVEMBER

Self-Loving Reason #11: Re-Charge Your Sex Drive!

If your libido feels like it's low on fuel, a nice masturbation session—or two, or three—might be just the injection you need. Stimulating yourself will get you feeling sexier because your entire body will respond: Your heart rate and blood flow increase. Your genitals and breasts swell and become more sensitive, your vaginal juices flow, and your skin flushes. Your brain releases all sorts of feel-good hormones. The erotic high from masturbation can last several hours.

Besides, the more orgasms you have, the more you'll want—and the more you'll get. Women who pleasure themselves regularly become aroused faster, have more orgasms, experience increased libido, have higher self-esteem, and have more satisfaction with sex and relationships. And just like any form of exercise, the more you do it, the better you'll become at it. In other words, your nervous system realizes, "Oh! We're doing this again!" and pops into gear faster each time. You'll have more pleasure with less effort.

Self-loving lets you recharge your libido in seconds flat. Most people can climax from masturbation in about four minutes. So do give yourself an orgasm a day. It could turn out to be a self-fulfilling prophecy!

NOVEMBER

Fitness for Your Pleasure

Hopefully, you've been doing your Kegels throughout the year (see January 7 and 8 if you need a review). As you know by now, these exercises are the single best way to tone and strengthen your pelvic floor muscle, also known as your PC (pubococcygeus) muscle. And a stronger PC muscle equals stronger, more intense orgasms. If you're the kind of gal who likes to accessorize her workout, you'll be glad to know that there are toys just for increasing sexual fitness—although you won't find them in any gym.

The Kegelcisor is a seven-inch stainless steel rod that resembles a barbell with little balls at either end and in the middle. It's marketed as a product for incontinence prevention, but what it does is give your PC muscle something to squeeze against when your man's love muscle isn't handy. The weight theoretically increases the resistance. Sex author Betty Dodson offers her own model, called "Betty's Barbell," and there's also a shorter, two-and-a-half-inch version called the Kegel Enhansor.

Another way to work your PC muscle is with a gadget called the vaginal weightlifting egg. Made of jade, onyx, or other semi-precious stones, these eggs are designed to be inserted into the vagina. A cord attached to the egg allows you to easily remove the egg, or add weights if necessary.

You don't need vaginal barbells to do your Kegels correctly, but they can certainly make your workout more interesting. And when you're ready for your cooldown—or warmup, as the case may be—your barbell is perfect for stimulating your G-spot!

NOVEMBER

Position of the Week: The Tenth Posture

Just because your man's on top in the missionary position, it doesn't mean he's in charge. The Tenth Posture of *The Perfumed Garden* lets you control the motion of the ocean. Lie on your back, reach over your head, and grab the headboard or rail of the bed. You could also brace yourself against the arm of your couch; in fact, the author suggests "a low divan." As your man enters you, clasp him tightly around the waist and hips with your legs. He then leans forward and grabs the headboard as well; he can also grip the edge of the bed with his toes. If you don't have a headboard, push against the wall.

Now the fun starts as *you* initiate the movements! He matches the rhythm of your thrusts as you push and pull against the headboard, almost in a seesaw motion. Squeeze his hips tightly with your legs for leverage. You could even order him to hold still as you move against him. This would be a great position in which to enact some naughty bondage fantasies. Who gets tied up? It's up to you!

NOVEMBER

More, More, More!

Another type of multiple orgasm is the sequential orgasm, a series of climaxes that follow each other anywhere from one to ten minutes apart, with only a slight drop in arousal in between. In one study, a woman reported having 134 orgasms in one hour! Varying the type of stimulation you're getting—such as following oral sex by intercourse—may be key to having these. After you've climaxed, change your position: Go from missionary to being on top, or rear entry from side-to-side. Or have your lover switch from thrusting inside you to massaging your clitoris, which can keep you enjoying those blissful orgasmic contractions every five seconds or so. You may find that your orgasms get stronger in intensity, or they may simply fade into a wonderful afterglow.

Remember, just because your body is capable of having several orgasms in a row doesn't mean you're going to want that many. Researcher Shere Hite found that most women are completely satisfied with one. When it comes to orgasms, it's quality, not quantity, that counts—and by quality, that doesn't mean that every orgasm has to rock your world. All that matters is that you enjoy the process. In fact, one of the best ways to ensure an orgasm is to do nothing. Stop trying and the orgasm, or several, may just come to you. As the thirteenth-century Sufi poet Rumi said:

> *"Observe the wonders as they occur around you. Don't claim them. Feel the artistry moving through and be silent."*

NOVEMBER

Dildos: The World's Oldest Sex Toys

For centuries, people have been pleasuring themselves with penis-like objects known commonly as dildos, derived from the Italian word *diletto*, or "delight." Representations of dildos have been found in 30,000-year-old Upper Paleolithic art, and appeared on Greek vase paintings in the fourth and fifth centuries B.C. Dildos have often been regarded as sacred objects. For example, in India, lingams (dildos) made of stone and ivory were used to represent the god Shiva. So when you buy a dildo for your pleasure, know that you're part of a long and historical tradition.

There's actually a physical reason for the dildo's popularity. When your body gets sexually aroused, your vagina balloons or "tents," and many women love the feeling of fullness and penetration. However, a dildo is *not* a penis substitute—it's a lovely toy to that allows you to penetrate yourself or your partner in different ways.

A quick definition: a dildo is any object you can insert in your vagina or bottom. If it vibrates, it's a vibrator, and not a dildo, although many dildos are hollow and can accommodate a battery-operated vibrating egg or bullet. Dildos come in a staggering variety of sizes, shapes, and colors to satisfy your every sensual mood. They're perfect for solo play because they put you in charge of the angle, depth, and speed of penetration—and they can be used creatively during partner sex as well! Dildos are fun, simple to use, and safe, and over the next few days, we'll talk about how to get the most out of yours.

NOVEMBER

Your Dildo Shopping List

Here are few simple questions that will help you pick the perfect dildo—or dildos—for your needs.

✦ **What do you plan to do with your toy?** To simulate intercourse, choose a traditional dildo, many of which resemble real penises. For G-spot stimulation, look for a dildo that's curved at the end. If you're going to use your dildo with a partner, consider a double-ended or harness-compatible dildo; the latter have a flared base.

✦ **What do you want it to feel like?** Dildos made of silicone or materials like cyberskin feel amazingly like real skin—they even warm to the touch. They're a little pricier, but many women consider the extra expense worth it. More affordable options are jelly rubber (known as "jellies") and latex. (Remember, porous toys require more care and cleaning.) If you think you'd like something rigid, acrylic and glass dildos come in beautiful curved, rippled, and smooth varieties.

✦ **What size do you want?** Most dildos come in diameters ranging from one-and-a-half to two inches. Don't underestimate the size of your aroused vagina, but don't let your eyes be bigger than your appetites. Use any current toys—fingers, your man's penis, cucumbers—as a guide. You can control how deeply you insert a dildo, but you can't change its width.

Finally, always apply lubricant to your dildo, no matter how aroused you are—two slippery surfaces are much better than one. You can make applying the lube part of your sensual ritual: Begin by wetting your toy with saliva, just as you would your man's member (what a way to practice your oral skills!), and then finish by anointing it with lube. Playtime!

NOVEMBER

Playtime with Your Pleasure Toys

What can you do with your dildo? Everything and anything that feels good, at your own pace, and in your own way. If you're just getting started, the key is to relax, breathe, and be gentle with yourself. Let your body's sensations guide you.

Here's a way to get acquainted with your new pleasure toy. First, get comfortable on your bed, leaning back on a chair or couch, or even on your pillow-covered floor. Lube up your toy, and begin caressing your vaginal lips with the lubed head, gliding it over your clitoris. Using either the dildo or your fingers to massage your love button will get your juices flowing enough to make penetration—if that's what's on the menu—even more sensuous.

When you're ready, begin gently penetrating your opening with the head of the dildo. If it's a realistic model, you might start by just dipping the glans inside. Tease yourself with short, slow strokes at first as your excitement builds, gradually building up to longer, deeper strokes. Get your PC muscle into the action, squeezing and relaxing in time with your thrusts as you imagine that you're milking your man's penis. Carry on until you can't stand it anymore!

NOVEMBER

The World's Best Aphrodisiac: Thoughtfulness

Want to *really* get your partner in the mood? Bear in mind that the special, thoughtful things you do for your lover work better than any pill or cream or fancy sexual technique. Liane, a project manager for a construction company, says that "The hottest thing a lover's ever done for me is arrange for a masseuse to come to the house, set up her table in front of the fireplace, and give me a two-hour massage. Afterwards I went straight to bed for a nap, and when I woke up I was *so* ready to make love to him. His thoughtfulness and consideration made me crazy with desire."

Your thoughtful gestures don't have to be elaborate. Amelia, a thirty-four-year-old financial services advisor, tells the following story: "During the last cold spell, my lover lay on my side of the bed to warm it up while I was getting ready for bed. When he told me what he was doing, my heart exploded with love, and it was the start to an amazing night of lovemaking."

Many sex experts point out that women in particular get turned on by feeling connected to their partner and feeling valued by him. That thoughtfulness works both ways. Your guy needs to know that you think he's special to you. Maybe you tape his favorite show when he has to work late. Or throw a surprise party for him. Or just bring him a cup of coffee when he's trying to finish that presentation for tomorrow's meeting. Thoughtfulness won't just win you brownie points—it will keep you connected, in love, and passionate about each other.

NOVEMBER

Room Service Begins at Home

When you really want to treat your partner, take a tip from the five-star hotels of the world. A Parisian friend of mine adopts this philosophy when he wants to pamper his lucky wife. "I indulge her with things a luxury hotel in Asia would do, such as spreading rose petals on the bed, buying her fine soaps and bath oils, or bringing her breakfast in bed with tangerine segments arranged like a flower, special china, and fine linen and silver," he says. "Having champagne in fine crystal flutes just for the hell of it makes an occasion *'la fête'!*"

As human beings, we love getting attentive treatment, no matter what our gender. "Every man I know loves to be pampered," says one friend. "That's why we're such hopeless wimps when we have a cold." Showing your lover how special you think he is out of the bedroom also translates into pleasure *in* the bedroom. "A sense of feeling appreciated makes lovemaking so much more extraordinary," says my friend Nanette. So one morning, make your man feel like he's woken up in the world's finest resort. Bring him his favorite breakfast and newspaper, give him a wonderful massage, and then crawl into bed with him. Now, *that's* room service!

NOVEMBER

Position of the Week: The Ascending Position

Unlike the male-focused *Perfumed Garden*, the *Ananga Ranga* of Kalyana Malla places great emphasis on ensuring that a woman achieve as much sexual satisfaction as her partner. In particular, the *Ananga Ranga* recommends woman-on-top positions for situations when "he, being exhausted, is no longer capable of muscular exertion, and when she is ungratified, being still full of the water of love."

The Ascending Position is a cross-legged position from the *Ananga Ranga* suggested for the woman "whose passion has not been gratified by previous copulation." With your man lying on his back, lower yourself onto his lingam, sitting in a cross-legged position as you "seize" him with your vagina. You can then move yourself up and down, or in any direction that gives you the stimulation that you need. You might even be able to reach your G-spot. This position leaves your hands free to massage your clitoris as well. Kalyana Malla comments that the woman "will derive great comfort" from this position. Try this position on a crisp fall evening, and you just might find out that he was right!

NOVEMBER

The Chakras: Putting It All Together

Sexual arousal automatically sends energy coursing through your chakras, and harnessing this energy can take your erotic bliss to new heights. Begin by sitting together in the classic Yab Yum sitting position, lowering yourself onto him and wrapping your legs around each other. Take a minute to stroke and kiss each other's face, hands, and skin, allowing yourselves to be wrapped in a cocoon of love. Open yourselves to your feelings of trust and intimacy.

Now, starting with your root chakra, imagine your energy centers opening one by one to form a channel that draws the energy up from your genitals and through each chakra, all the way into your crown. You can use several methods to help you visualize this. For example, you could chant or hum mantras (consult a Web site like www.schooloftantra.com for the appropriate one) as you visualize the energy moving through you. You could also imagine each chakra being filled with its associated color: Red for the root center; orange, the sex center; yellow, the solar plexus; green, the heart center; blue, the throat center; indigo, the third eye; and violet, the crown. Throughout this process, focus on your breathing, allowing it to slow down and deepen your arousal.

My friend Kim, a forty-three-year-old photographer, finds that bringing her energy up in this manner—either alone or with a partner—allows sensation to spread throughout her body, bringing her to a full-body orgasm. "If you choose not to climax," she says, "you'll exist for several hours in a heightened state." Try it sometime!

NOVEMBER

Breathe into Orgasms

Your breathing patterns have a strong impact on your orgasms. Faster breathing increases your excitement, while deep breathing and exhaling through your mouth in time with your release can give you more intense climaxes. Deep breathing also sends more oxygen to your muscles, including the ones in your genitals. In fact, if you have trouble achieving orgasms, try changing your breathing pattern. Instead of holding your breath, try inhaling and exhaling deeply. Or match your breathing to your partner's, which will strengthen the bond between you.

Breathing from your diaphragm—the muscle that separates your chest and abdominal cavity—helps as well. To practice this, exhale forcefully and bring your belly up at the same time, forcing the air out (this is similar to the Breath of Fire described on July 25). You should feel your diaphragm contracting. Try this during an orgasm and see if you don't have a super-charged climax.

Many of us breathe shallowly from our chests when we're stressed. If, after a hard day, you feel anxious or tense before sex, relax yourself and raise your sexual energy by breathing deeply from your stomach instead of your chest. Inhale, pulling your stomach in as far as you can. Exhale, pushing your stomach out, and count to five. You'll be more energetic, more sensitive to pleasure, and able to slow down so that you can really enjoy the sensual feelings.

NOVEMBER

Crossing That Bridge When You Come (Together)

Your body is a marvelously programmable instrument. If you want to expand your sexual repertoire, try the "bridge" technique, so called because it allows you to build a bridge from your tried-and-true way of climaxing to new ways of reaching sexual nirvana. Ask your man to massage your clitoris during intercourse, or do it yourself. As you feel yourself getting ready to climax, stop rubbing your love button and focus solely on his thrusts and the feeling of him inside you as you go over the top. Over the next weeks or months, stop stimulating your clitoris a little sooner. Soon, the feeling of your man inside you will trigger your orgasm. For variation, have him stimulate you orally, and then switch to intercourse right before you come.

The bridge technique certainly isn't meant replace your other methods of achieving the Big O, nor does it imply that there's anything wrong with a clitoral orgasm, which is what most women experience. But it may give you a better chance of having a simultaneous climax with your honey, especially if you work to recognize each other's verbal and physical arousal cues as well.

NOVEMBER

Sagittarius, the Archer

If you or your man were born between November 22 and December 21, you fall under the sign of Sagittarius, the archer. Sagittarians are the warm-hearted, playful adventurers of the zodiac. They're friendly, fun-loving, honest (sometimes brutally so), and intellectual. Optimistic by nature, a typical Sagittarian always believes that everything will turn out fine.

Your Sagittarian man loves active, lusty, no-holds-barred sex. If you're looking for someone to last all night—after a full day of hiking or downhill skiing—this is your man. In fact, Sagittarians love sex in the great outdoors. Remember that Sagittarius is represented by a centaur—half man, half beast. Anything that takes you back to nature will get those primordial juices flowing. There's science to back this up as well. After you've been in the sun fifteen minutes or more, your brain starts releasing serotonin, the feel-good hormone, so if you live somewhere with cold and rainy Novembers, by all means plan a getaway to somewhere sunny.

To a Sagittarian, physical exertion equals foreplay. Work out for an hour or so before you get busy. Vigorous exercise will get your blood flowing and get you in peak aerobic shape, which is great preparation for intense orgasms. Research has also shown that working out increases sexual responsiveness, so challenge your man to a game of tennis. Race him down a double-black-diamond mountain. Take him out for a wild night of dancing. Then get him home and out of his clothes for a wild night of lovemaking.

NOVEMBER

More Ways to Up Your Odds of Ecstasy

If you want to increase your chances of climaxing in the missionary position, try these variations. Have your man raise himself onto his elbows or hands, putting more pressure on your clitoris. Or pull your knees into your chest and spread them apart, making a V of your legs. This will allow his pubic bone to grind against your vulva and clitoris while his penis rubs against your G-spot. If you drape your legs over his shoulder, you lengthen your vagina so that he can penetrate you more deeply and increase the pressure both inside and out.

Another trick is to close your legs together tightly and have him put his legs outside yours from a kneeling or lying position. This increases the friction on both of you in delightful ways. If you're on top, you can do almost the same thing: Stretch out on top of him so your legs are straddling his thighs, then push yourself up onto your hands to arch your back (like the Cobra pose in yoga). This puts your clitoris in direct contact with his pubic bone.

And while we're at it, another woman-on-top move: Try rubbing your clitoris against him, then planting your feet or knees on either side of him and swiveling your hips, almost as if you were letting him stir your juices with his staff.

Here's an internal trick that you can try from any position: Bear down on him with your PC muscles, as though you were trying to push him out. By doing so, you'll push your G-spot closer to your vaginal opening, and thus his member, making ecstatic contact a sure thing.

NOVEMBER

Multiple Orgasms for Him

Multiple male orgasms happen in one of two ways. The first, which mostly happens in younger men, is when a man has more than one orgasm, including ejaculation, with a very brief refractory period between erections. The second and more common type occurs when a man trains himself to have an orgasm without ejaculation and without losing his erection. One method your man can use to do this is to play with his arousal level. Have him stimulate himself until he's on the verge of climaxing, then back off for up to twenty seconds before he starts up again.

The second key is a well-toned PC muscle. Yes, men can do their Kegels, too! The drill is the same as for you: Squeeze, hold, and release. If you're feeling playful, drape a washcloth over his erect member and have him try to move it up and down with his penis. As you might guess, a buff male PC muscle makes sex all the more exciting—imagine holding completely still while he moves his member inside your aroused vagina.

With practice, your man may be able to combine his newly fit PC muscle with his awareness of his own arousal levels to prevent himself from ejaculating when he climaxes. He'll still have all the wonderful sensations of an orgasm, including rapid heart rates, muscle contractions and the feeling of release—he just won't ejaculate. Tantric sex practitioners believe that translates to more time to connect spiritually and physically, while Taoists believe that controlling ejaculation conserves sexual energy. (However, holding back from ejaculation too often could cause prostate problems, so don't make it a habit.) Whatever your philosophy, multiple male orgasms hold out the potential of more bliss for both of you.

NOVEMBER

Position of the Week: The Tail of the Ostrich

So you're in yoga class, diligently practicing your Downward Dog and forward bends, when suddenly, you have a slightly scandalous thought. "What would it be like to have sex in this pose?" you wonder. Well, the *Perfumed Garden* position called The Tail of the Ostrich might just help you find out. As you lie on your back, pretend that you're about to do a shoulderstand, but instead of you raising your legs into position, your man kneels in front of you and lifts your legs until only your head and shoulders are still resting on the bed. Twine your legs around his neck as he—carefully—enters you. The author says that the man then "seizes and sets into motion the buttocks of the woman." Whatever he does, he should do it slowly.

Here's where yoga experience comes in handy. As in a yoga shoulderstand, you might put some blankets under your shoulders. Be very careful to keep your neck bent (keep your eyes focused on him or on your bellybutton). Don't turn your head from side-to-side. Press your hands into the back of your torso to support yourself. He can also hold your hips.

Don't stay in this position very long, but it could be fun to experiment with. You might try it with your upper body hanging off the bed or couch—the blood rushing to your head could produce some interesting sensations!

NOVEMBER

Give Thanks for Sensual Gifts

What are you thankful for this Thanksgiving? How about making a sexual gratitude list? After all, isn't the fact that our bodies can give us such intense and utter bliss something for which we should be thankful? What a gift!

Think about all the things you like about your sexuality. You might be thankful for the way your nipples respond to touch, or the delicious orgasms you have with your favorite vibrator. Maybe you love how you look when you're aroused, or the skill you've developed at driving your man to distraction with your mouth. Count your erotic blessings!

By now you know that one of the secrets to great relationships is taking the time to appreciate each other. Maybe you've got a partner who's willing to do whatever it takes to please you in bed. Or maybe he's always telling you how much he loves your butt or legs, making you reconsider your decision to worry incessantly about that particular body part. One of my male friends tells me, "I've heard it said that women like to be appreciated for who they are, while men prefer to be appreciated for what they do. I think this is largely true." So today, be generous with those two words that everyone—especially your sweetie—loves to hear: Thank you!

NOVEMBER

Crescent of Pleasure

You can send your pleasure sky-high by stimulating what's known as the "orgasmic crescent," an area that includes the clitoris, the clitoral network that extends into the body, the urethra and the urethral sponge, and the G-spot (the spongy tissue that swells when you become aroused). Next time your lover goes down south on you, ask him to pay attention to your clitoral tip, urethral opening, and G-spot all at once with his mouth and hands. Then hang on!

Speaking of your urethra (the opening between your clitoris and vagina), it's not just the place from which you pee. Because it's surrounded by the body of the clitoris, and farther up, the urethral sponge (which contains your G-spot), some women can have powerful orgasms when their "U-spot" is stimulated with firm pressure from a tongue or hand. Other women just find this annoying and unpleasant. But here's a way to see if this is one of your hot spots: Ask your man to wrap his lower lip over his bottom teeth and press up firmly while he's massaging your clitoris with his mouth or tongue. Stimulating this area can be nice after you've had your orgasm, especially if your clitoris isn't happy with continued direct stimulation. Just make sure he's clean-shaven!

NOVEMBER

In the Zone

The G-spot isn't the only attraction in your tunnel of love. The Anterior Fornix Erogenous (AFE) zone is located on the front wall of your vagina, about halfway between your cervix and your G-spot. Studies have shown pressure on the "A-spot" can produce stronger orgasms, and more of them. To find it, slide one or two fingers into your vagina until you reach your G-spot. Keep going, and you'll touch your cervix, which will feel something like the end of your nose. Right between your cervix and the G-spot is your AFE zone. Have your lover move his fingers in a circular motion inside you, or thrust into you from behind while you're on your hands and knees.

You might find that your cervix is also sensitive to pressure. Many women have intense, all-over orgasms when their cervixes are stimulated during deep penetration by a long dildo or their man's thrusting penis. To find out if you're one of them, hop on top of him facing his feet to allow maximum penetration.

Another spot that responds to pressure is the cul-de-sac behind the cervix that's created when your uterus lifts and your upper vagina balloons during sexual arousal. Try lifting your legs up when you're in the missionary position to help him reach this area.

Remember, everyone's different, and stimulating these spots may send you over the moon or leave you decidedly land-locked. Regardless, it always pays to learn about your body's geography. Happy exploring!

NOVEMBER

Physical Moves for Maximum Bliss

To get all the ecstasy you can, it pays not to be *too* relaxed. Bear in mind that an orgasm is the release of muscle tension, so you've got to have some to begin with. The adrenaline coursing through your veins focuses your mind and makes you ultra-sensitive, so think about the delicious mixture of anxiety and excitement when you're with a new lover. You can recreate this feeling even in long-term relationships. Next time you're knocking boots with your man, add some muscle tension by flexing your thighs and clenching your butt. This increases the blood flow to your pelvic area, which swells your clitoris and gets your vaginal juices flowing.

Another trick is to press down on your lower abdomen or squeeze those muscles during sex, which massages your inner clitoris. Remember that your clitoris is more than just a delightful knob. It actually consists of about nine inches of erectile tissue, so make the most of it. One way to do this when you're on top is to lean back so his penis pushes on your vagina's front wall. Meanwhile, massage your clitoris and nipples. He'll enjoy the view, and you'll enjoy the bliss!

NOVEMBER

Slow Down and Savor Each Other

Just because the days are getting shorter doesn't mean your lovemaking has to be. Here are a few ways to draw out the exquisite agony of sensual bliss:

+ If you're in the missionary position or on top, stretch out your legs alongside his. This will make his thrusts shallower. (Be careful with this one: The most sensitive nerve endings are in the head of the penis and the outer third of the vagina. Shallow thrusts could send him over the edge.)

+ If you start getting too close to climax, distract each other. Don't get up and answer the phone, just slow down what you're doing, talk, or do whatever you need to put the brakes on.

+ Move in slow motion. Do everything in twice the time it would normally take you, focusing on your breathing, movements, and motion.

+ Stop what you're doing for a moment—both of you—and savor the feeling of his penis inside you. This is a sex therapy technique called "vaginal containment" that was originally designed to help with premature ejaculation.

+ Lean away from each other. First, you sit on top of him, then both of you lean back and put your weight on your elbows or hands. You can put a stack of pillows behind your backs if that's more comfortable.

When you slow sex down, you'll become aware of pleasures you never noticed when you were going at it fast and furious. When you finally do climax, the results will be worth the wait.

CHAPTER TWELVE

DECEMBER

"In seed time learn, in harvest teach, in winter enjoy."
—*William Blake (1757-1827), British poet, painter,
engraver, and mystic*

As the year draws to a close, this month's tips take on a festive flair! Yes, it's the season of gift-giving, so why not give the gift of ecstasy to yourself or your man? You'll learn how to heat up those cold winter nights by driving your partner wild in bed, or how to relax after a long day of gift-shopping with a leisurely, delicious G-spot orgasm.

This month will also be a time for you to take stock of your sensual year with an inventory of lessons learned, and likes and dislikes. It's time to start planning *next year's* list of Sensual Resolutions!

There's some debate about this month's birth flower. Some consider it to be *holly*, which the Victorians used to represent foresight, the ability to think ahead. Others say that it's the *narcissus*, considered to be both a symbol of prosperity and a sign of self-love. You could decorate your house with both to represent your newfound ability to see good things to come. The choice is yours.

This month's birthstone, *turquoise*, is also a symbol of prosperity. Find a way to incorporate either the color or the stone itself into your life to represent your hopes for a prosperous and sensual New Year ahead!

DECEMBER

Be a Tease—to Yourself

If you want a more intense orgasm, don't hurry. Instead, tease yourself mercilessly. Bring yourself to the brink of an orgasm and stay there for as long as possible, then back off a little and switch to a less sensitive area for a while. For example, you might bring yourself close to an orgasm by massaging your clitoris, then move to your inner labia. Each time, your arousal will mount a little more. Savor it. Note the sensations. Prolong your pleasure as though it were the best five-course meal you've ever had. When you finally do take yourself over the edge, you'll have one stupendous climax. Why does this work? An orgasm is the release of tension, so it stands to reason that the more tension you have in your body, the better the release.

You can give your lover permission to tease you, too, but it takes some communication. First of all, you have to get yourself in the right mental state. Give yourself permission to focus on yourself—don't worry, it will be his turn soon enough. Let him begin stimulating you by your preferred method. (He doesn't have ESP, so you'll have to tell him what that method is and fill him in on the whole teasing thing.) Since you're going to be drawing things out, you might want him to use his hands (rather than his mouth), and lots of lube. When you feel yourself getting close, ask him to shift his attention to another part of your genitals. Ride the roller coaster a few times before you let him take you off the tracks and straight to heaven.

DECEMBER

Position of the Week: Two Fishes

In Taoist thought, two twin and opposing forces animate the universe and are constantly striving for balance: Yin, which is feminine, and Yang, which represents the masculine. During sex, men and women exchange these energies, which become most potent during climax. In this school of thought, sex is not about romance or spirituality, but about improving one's health, developing character, and living a longer life. In fact, Taoist physicians concluded over two thousand years ago that sex is necessary to physical, mental, and spiritual well-being.

The seventh-century Taoist pillow book *T'ung Hsüan Tzu* by physician Li T'ung Hsüan portrays twenty-six positions for lovemaking. The Two Fishes position seems to evoke the Yin-Yang symbol itself, a circle divided into two black-and-white curving, fish-shaped sections. Lie on your sides facing each other, your legs together. After he slips inside you, you lift your legs onto his as though you were a fish wrapping its tail around her mate.

This position was designed for men with especially long penises, but even so, it allows only shallow penetration, which can be fun in itself! He could also easily caress your sex with the tip of his member, teasing and preparing you for deeper penetration to come.

DECEMBER

Lengthening His Pleasure

Is your man occasionally a little quick on the draw? Here's a way to slow him down, give him a truly heavenly sexual experience, and extend the pleasure for both of you. Just as you teased yourself on December 1 in order to enjoy a more potent climax, today you're going to help him raise his orgasmic threshold by bringing him close to, but not into, his orgasm several times. While lovingly stroking his member with your hand, ask him to rate his arousal on a scale of one to ten, with ten being the Big O. When he says he's reached a three or four, slow down until his arousal ebbs a little, then start up again until he's at a six or eight. Slow down. Repeat. (Hint: you can always get an idea of when he's about to come by watching his scrotum. When his testicles pull up into his body, he's very, very close.)

Do this for about fifteen minutes, until you finally take him all the way to a perfect ten. Chances are that when he finally does come, he'll have an orgasm that will rock his world.

The key is to help him learn when he's at the point of no return—technically known as "ejaculatory inevitability." If he goes over it once or twice, no big deal. The idea isn't to deny him sensation, it's to help him grow familiar with and enjoy different levels of arousal. After a while, you can work this technique into your lovemaking, too. You'll learn to read his symptoms of arousal, and you can both pace yourselves to a rollicking climax.

DECEMBER

Orgasm Busters

Having trouble reaching orgasm? There are several factors that can keep you from going over the edge to ecstasy:

+ **Antidepressants.** Selective serotonin reuptake inhibitors (SSRIs) like Prozac can decrease sensation, make it harder for you to achieve orgasms, and affect your libido. **Solution:** Talk to your doctor about your dosage or alternate medications, like Wellbutrin.

+ **Stress.** When you're stressed, your body reduces its production of sex hormones. Basically, your body isn't going to be making you feel sexy when it thinks you need to survive. **Solution:** Find ways to calm your mind. Take a walk or a hot bath. Do yoga, or meditate. In bed, focus on relaxing and letting go.

+ **Sleep deprivation.** Getting less sleep can affect your libido. People who suffer from chronic insomnia have higher levels of stress hormones in their blood. **Solution:** Get seven to eight hours rest.

+ **Alcohol.** Sure, a drink or two may relax you, but drinking a lot of booze constricts your blood vessels, meaning that less blood flows to your naughty bits. It also interferes with sex hormone production. **Solution:** If you're going to drink, keep it to a glass (or half a glass) of red wine, which does have several health benefits.

+ **Hormonal imbalances.** Scientists are looking at whether low levels of testosterone decrease sexual functioning. **Solution:** Talk to your doctor about having your levels tested.

+ **Fear.** You're afraid you'll catch an STD (sexually transmitted disease) or get pregnant. **Solution:** Use a condom!

A final problem: Putting too much pressure on yourself. If you don't climax every time you masturbate or make love, don't sweat it. Make pleasure your goal, and your orgasm just one possible and delightful outcome.

DECEMBER

Clothing for Your (and His) Eyes Only

Are you making your holiday wish list? If so, put erotic clothing at the top of the list. Ask him to buy you the sexiest piece of lingerie he can find. Give him the Victoria's Secret catalog for inspiration. Tell him that when he sees you wearing his gift—peeking out from your cleavage or the top of your jeans—it will be your signal that the two of you are going to get busy later.

Now, maybe sexy lingerie isn't your thing, or his. Some men much prefer the sight of naked skin to satin and lace, God bless 'em. So have him buy you whatever he finds particularly sexy, and use that as your signal. The idea is that you have a secret sign to each other, so that if he sees you wearing that certain pair of earrings, he knows you want him to bend you over the couch and ravish you from behind.

If you aren't in a relationship right now, go out and buy something sexy *for yourself.* Something that makes you feel like you're the hottest thing on two legs. So what if you're the only person who knows you're wearing it? If it makes you feel sexy, that's all that matters. Wear a satin camisole under a sweater, garters and stockings under your business suit, or a push-up bra under your favorite T-shirt. Look for fabrics that caress your skin and make you feel like the sex goddess you really are, inside and out!

DECEMBER

Encourage Mental Foreplay

Put your erotic imagination, and his, to work for you by talking about sex, sexy things, and the sexy things you're wearing when he's least able to do anything about it. The idea is to get his mind (and yours, too) on an X-rated track and keep it there until you're alone. Here's a move suggested by my friend Mark: "At dinner one night, my girlfriend told me in detail what she was wearing under her outfit. She also took the opportunity to discuss future lingerie purchases as well. Then, at the end of dinner, she excused herself and went to the ladies' room. When she came back, she slipped her panties into my hand and gave me a kiss. I could hardly wait for the check to arrive."

The idea is to get him thinking about what you look like naked, making both of you so hot and bothered that you'll be dying to get your hands on each other. Let's be honest: When you meet someone attractive, don't you find yourself, however briefly, trying to picture what he looks like without his clothes? If you don't, you should! You'll give yourself the material for a very erotic fantasy to enjoy later by yourself, back in the comfort of your own private boudoir.

DECEMBER

Sex in Tight Spaces

It's the holiday season, and you and your man are out doing your shopping when the mood overtakes you. Question is, how do you make all the right moves when you don't have much room? Assuming you can find some privacy, standing positions are your best bet. Brace yourself against a wall and stand with your feet about hip width or more apart. He should stand with his feet between yours, bend his knees and enter you from below, holding onto your hips for support. On a staircase, stand one step above him. In a dressing room, have him sit on a bench or sturdy chair while you perch on top of him (be careful, as many department stores use two-way mirrors).

It helps if your anatomy is conducive to having sex in any position. My friend Eve says, "The hottest thing I've ever done with a lover—having sex outside standing at some corner on a random street—was only possible because he had a long penis." If you're outside and lucky enough to find a secluded place, here's a way to keep your clothes from getting dirty—have him squat on his heels while you sit on his upper thighs.

Dress for success while you're at it. It helps if he goes "commando-style" (without underwear), but if not, simply pull his erection out of his shorts. Hopefully, you're wearing your thinnest thong. Just pull it to one side, and away you go!

DECEMBER

Party Time

Turn a boring holiday party into an occasion for a daring tryst. Sneak off into your host's bedroom, bathroom, or a closet for some quick and furtive lovemaking. If you've got room, he can kneel while you lie in front of him, your knees pulled to your chest. Or brace yourself against the wall or bathroom counter. At the office party, lock an office door and back a chair up against a wall, or lie back on the desk. If you're at a restaurant, no one will think anything if the bathroom door's locked for five minutes. (Just make sure there's not a line.) You'll return to the festivities with a big smile and glowing skin.

Of course, when it comes to private activity in public places, you don't have to go all the way. My friend Andrew says that he's had a girlfriend almost bring him to the point of climax by teasing him through his clothes at a restaurant, under the cover of the white linen tablecloth. You can use either your fingers or your toes. "Once he's erect," he advises, "subtly tap the tip of his erect penis with your fingers throughout dinner. You may even be able to bring him to an orgasm." Try this, and your man won't want to linger over coffee.

DECEMBER

Position of the Week: A Silkworm Spinning a Cocoon

The writers of Chinese pillow books embellished their instructions with evocative language to describe the human sexual organs and the sexual act itself. For example, the penis is referred to as the Jade Stem, Coral Stem, Turtle Head, and Heavenly Dragon Pillar. Names for the female genitalia include Coral Gate, Jade Gate, Open Peony Blossom, and Jade Pavilion. The clitoris and its surrounding area are called the Pearl on the Jade Step and Jewel Terrace.

The names for the sexual positions themselves are rich in natural imagery, with man-on-top positions falling under the basic posture known as Intimate Union. In the beautifully named A Silkworm Spinning a Cocoon, you lie on your back and spread your thighs as far as you can. Wrap your legs tightly around him so that you can pull yourself up and down in time with his thrusts. By exposing your Pearl on the Jade Step to stimulation by his Coral Stem, you may not only experience what the Taoists called Bursting of the Clouds, you may also find yourself sailing high above them!

DECEMBER

Getaway Surprise

If your man likes surprises (and who doesn't!), get his engines revving by whisking him away to a special dinner at his favorite restaurant, a club to hear his favorite band, or even a weekend out of town. Keep your destination unknown until the very last minute. "Being kidnapped is really nice," says my friend Tim, a graduate student. "I love being abducted for a nice dinner and then getting molested back home. A spontaneous cool night out that you planned ahead of time can be great. Just make sure it doesn't conflict with plans I already have!"

By taking the initiative to plan dates or weekends out of town (not to mention giving him the spontaneous "pick-me-up" blowjob), show your man you care about him and want to keep the relationship fresh and alive. It's especially important if there are kids in the picture, since it allows you to focus on your needs as a couple.

One friend of mine surprised his wife by announcing over champagne on New Year's Day that he was checking her into a fancy hotel just outside of town and coming back for her two days later. "She luxuriated in the room service, amazing pool and spa, sleeping late (impossible at home with our two-year-old son), reading, and going for walks," he said. "I joined her for dinner on Saturday night and felt like her lover creeping away as the midnight hour approached." You could adapt this to your own needs by sending your man off to your favorite hotel. Tell him you'll meet him later, then appear at the door wearing nothing but a coat!

DECEMBER

Sensational Sensations

Don't forget that the skin can be a marvelous sex toy. Experiment with different sensations as part of your sensual play. Blindfold him and drag different textures across his skin—satin, fur, the bristles of a natural-hair brush, a silk scarf, your fingernails. And don't forget the ice: Make like the movie *9½ Weeks* and trail ice cubes across his overheated body. Slide them over his testicles and play with the entrance to his secret hole. (Be careful about slipping ice inside, however, in consideration of delicate tissues.) If you've been playing around with a little light S&M, imagine how ice will feel applied to a freshly spanked bottom.

Imagine, too, how ice would feel alternated with something hot—like wax. Yes, candles aren't just for sensual boudoir lighting! Tease him with some temperature play, but be sure to use plain paraffin candles, as colored, scented, and beeswax candles burn at a higher temperature. Start by holding the candle high above his body—at least a few feet, because the wax will cool as it falls—and let it drip on him, one drip at a time. "This is very intense and very erotic," says my friend Kyle. By the way, unless you want him to understand what a bikini wax is like, drip the wax on his less-hairy parts. *Never* drip wax on his face or genitals. This is supposed to be fun torture, not bad torture.

You can gradually move the candle closer, but test it occasionally on your own skin so you can ensure it's not too hot. Who gets to peel off the dried wax? That's up to you.

DECEMBER

Self-Loving Reason #12: Better Partner Sex!

If you know how to make yourself hot and bothered, your chances of having sizzling sex with your partner increase exponentially. Think about it. If self-loving puts you in touch with your body, teaches you about your sexual response, increases your libido and allows you to achieve more orgasms on a regular basis, how can your man *not* benefit? You'll be an excited, willing, and creative lover—something every man craves. You know what turns you on, and you can show him exactly what it is. He doesn't need to guess. He doesn't have to worry that he's not pleasing you. Most guys *want* directions on how to satisfy you. You can give him the keys to the kingdom because you know exactly where they are!

What's more, when you're comfortable with arousing yourself, you can give him a show he'll never forget. Men are visual creatures—they love to watch. And they love, love, love, seeing you turn yourself on (it also helps them pick up pointers). You can also show him sensuous tricks he never knew existed. While your guy may not know what Kegels are, he'll sure appreciate them when your PC muscle, toned by regular self-induced climaxes, flutters on his member during climax.

Finally, don't forget that sharing your most intimate needs with your partner is a deeply intimate act. You're showing each other your most out-of-control, ecstatic sexual selves. Being open and vulnerable with each other is what allows intimacy to flourish, partners to become soulmates, and good sex to become extraordinary.

DECEMBER

G-Spot Gifts

If you're looking for new ways to pleasure your G-spot, try a toy designed especially for that purpose. Look for slender dildos or vibrators curved to caress you in exactly the right place, and, in the case of vibrators, to buzz against the front wall of your love canal. If you're still discovering your G-spot, some models feature wider heads that cover more area. For women who want to double their fun, there are even G-spot vibrators that sport nubbed clitoral stimulators. You'll find G-spot vibes made of many of the same materials as other toys, such as jelly rubber, plastic, or vinyl. You'll also find silicone or vinyl G-spot attachments for your Hitachi Magic Wand. Choose a firmer material if your G-spot craves firm pressure, or softer materials if you like a gentler touch.

To get the most out of your G-spot vibrator, use it in the positions that offer the most G-spot stimulation: Woman on top or rear entry. Tuck your well-lubed vibrator in between two firm pillows or even better, two couch cushions. Lower yourself onto it while imagining it's your man's straining erection, or kneel on your bed and slide it into yourself from behind. (I'm sure you man will be glad to lend a hand if needed.) Or simply lie back, and adjust your toy until you find the angle that presses against your goddess spot.

By the way, a G-spot vibrator can double as the perfect prostate stimulator for your man. During lovemaking or oral sex, ease the well-lubed tip about three inches into his bottom, and buzz him to ecstasy.

DECEMBER

Pleasure at Your Fingertips

With fingertip vibrators, you can let your fingers do the walking. The most popular is the Fukuoku 9000, a battery vibrator with little rubber sleeves that fit right on the tip of your finger. Powered by watch batteries, the Fukuoku does away with the need for battery packs and cords. You'll hardly know you're wearing anything, which makes it a great addition to either solo play or partner sex. Slip your vibrating finger between your bodies to tease your clitoris and the base of his penis. Trail your finger over his testicles and down to his perineum. Let your imagination go wild!

To rev up your sensations even more, check out the Fukuoku Power pack, which consists of three fingertip vibes! You control the speed with a battery pack that attaches to your wrist. The beauty of this model is that you can glide your hand all over your skin—or his—for a wonderful massage. Run your fingers over your scalp, breasts, nipples, stomach, and sensitive inner thighs. Wearing this turbo-charged pleasure toy, you might feel a little bit like the Bionic Woman. In fact, with this toy, you might be able to last all night!

DECEMBER

Don't Just Vibrate—Eroscillate!

If you like to be on the cutting edge of technology, try the Eroscillator, a vibrator that looks somewhat like an electric toothbrush. You have to hand it to the makers of this product for not hiding behind coy euphemisms: The Web site, www.eroscillator.com, states proudly that the Eroscillator is "the first device designed exclusively for sexual excitement of the female genitalia." So how does this clever gadget, the product of Swiss engineering and ten years of research, offer women "exciting, immensely satisfying orgasms with little or no effort?" By oscillating—not vibrating—against your clitoris at 3,600 steady oscillations per minute. The drawback is the price—you'll pay about $100 for the "entry-level" model.

If you're not sure you want to plunk down that much change, a ready-made vibrator may be as close as your bathroom sink. Did you know that your electric toothbrush can be drafted for erotic purposes? Just cover the bristles with a condom or plastic wrap, or use the back of the tip. Wash well after use. Whiter teeth, fresh breath, and erotic bliss—what more could you ask?

DECEMBER

Position of the Week: Mandarin Ducks

Mandarin ducks are said to form such a strong attachment to their partners that, if separated, they pine for each other and die of loneliness. As a result, practitioners of *feng shui*, the Chinese art of placement, often use them as they symbolize love and conjugal fidelity. (Sadly, these beautiful birds are becoming quite rare in their native eastern Asia.) The Taoist position Mandarin Ducks may get its name from the mating of these loyal creatures. It's great for those of us who like to spoon in bed, or be awakened with our lovers inside us!

Lie on your sides with your back to your man, his knees tucked into yours as he enters you from behind. Prop your heads on pillows for support. If you don't mind mixing sexual philosophies, you can bring some Tantric practices into play by arranging your bodies so that his heart chakra lines up with yours. If it's comfortable, he can slide his arm under your neck and rest his hand on your third eye (the crown chakra). Synchronize your breathing and imagine energy flowing from his heart to yours. Let any tension or fears you have melt away as you feel his love envelop you.

DECEMBER

Send a Tingle Up His Spine

It's a cold winter night, and you're snuggled next to your honey in front of the fireplace, sipping a nightcap, and staring into each other's eyes. Did you know that your glass of liqueur can warm more than just your tummy? Take a sip of brandy or peppermint schnapps and run your tongue around his lips. Then slowly move down his chest, leaving a minty cool trail across his skin, all the way down to his naughty bits. The sensation will make him shiver with pleasure.

With a little advance preparation, you can draft some cinnamon or mint mouthwash for a similar purpose. Take a small amount into your mouth—just enough so that you won't accidentally swallow it—and as you slip your mouth over him, let the mouthwash drip down his shaft. This move is known as a "tingler." There's no doubt that it will make him tingle with joy!

NOTE: If you like playing with sensations, you might be tempted to slap a little Tiger Balm, BenGay, or Icy Hot on your sensitive regions thinking that the cool, then hot sensation will feel kind of neat. It *won't*. A friend of mine who wants to remain nameless accidentally touched his unit after applying BenGay to a sore shoulder. "It was unbelievably painful," he says with a wince. So unless your man specifically requests this kind of treatment, use these types of ointments on your major muscle groups, and instead, look for products made for sensual purpose, like the edible Kama Sutra Oils of Love or Pleasure Balm.

DECEMBER

String of Pearls

During the holiday season, a beautiful string of pearls adds class and elegance to any outfit, and sensual delights to any erotic encounter. Lubricate a long string of costume pearls (real pearls don't like lube, nor does the string connecting them) and his waiting erection. Then wrap the pearls around him, taking care not to scratch him with the clasp. Once you've adorned his rod, begin to stroke him in a luxurious up-and-down motion with one or both hands.

You can also use your pearls to give yourself a treat. Roll the strand down to the bottom of his shaft and mount him, rubbing yourself against the tiny spheres. Or unfurl the necklace, slip it into your vagina, and pull the beads out one by one up and over your throbbing clitoris.

Another type of pearl necklace you've probably already heard about was mentioned on *Sex in the City*. Lie on your back with him straddling your waist. Fondle whatever you can reach as he pleasures himself to his heart's content. Egg him on with whatever moans and naughty comments you think make him hot. If he likes, you can even take over with some of your finely honed manual techniques. When he climaxes, direct his love juice onto your neck and upper chest (hence the name). They may not sell this kind of necklace at Saks, but he'll think you've given him one incredible gift.

HISTORICAL NOTE: Today is the birthday of Betty Grable (1916-73), the American actress who was known as the "pin-up" girl of World War II. At one point, her legs were insured for a million dollars!

DECEMBER

Your Body and His: New Frontiers

When you're getting frisky with your man, don't head straight below the belt. As we discussed on April 27, your bodies are sensual playgrounds from head to toe. Don't forget his underarms, the location of an amazing amount of nerve endings. To drive him wild, nuzzle or lick him here before he applies deodorant, or stroke him lightly up his sides. "This will make him go crazy," says one friend, who follows this advice to great effect with his own boyfriends. Besides, it may just turn you on, too—one study found that the natural pheromones here can send you into sexual overdrive.

While you're in the vicinity, move to the end of his arms. Good finger sucking shows him what you can do with your mouth, hinting at pleasures to come. Don't be delicate. Starting with his thumb, put the whole finger in your mouth, and Hoover away. Finish by tracing your tongue over his palm, then guide his wet hand to his member, or better yet, your breasts and the delicious wetness between your legs.

DECEMBER

Foot Reflexology for Lovers

After a long day of shopping or an evening of holiday parties, there's absolutely nothing more relaxing than a long foot massage. Besides, tending to your lover's aching feet is one of the most tender and nurturing things you can do for him. To get started, have him lie back on a couch or a pile of pillows, or, if you're giving each other foot massages at the same time, set yourselves up at opposite ends of a couch or bed.

You might start by soaking his feet in a bowl or tub of warm, scented water. Then gently dry his feet with a soft towel. Don't miss the area between the toes! Pour some massage oil or foot cream on your hands to warm it, and then begin massaging his feet. Do one foot at a time, starting softly, and gradually increasing your pressure. Use your thumb to press in long, deep strokes up the sole of his foot; use lighter strokes over his instep and sole. Stroke from the center of the foot out to the edge. Work your way out to his toes, checking in with him frequently to make sure you're not causing him any pain. When you reach his toes, pull gently but firmly from the base to the tip, starting from his little toe. Hold his ankle in one hand and rotate his foot with the other.

Getting a foot massage soothes both body and mind. It may be just the thing you need to help you relax and get in the mood for more stimulating activities!

DECEMBER

Celebrate the Winter Solstice

For thousands of years, cultures all over the world have observed the Winter Solstice, the longest night of the year, as a cause for celebration because after today, the days once again start getting longer. In Iran, this night is called *Shab-e Yalda*, or "night of birth," and it marks the eve of the birth of Mithra, the sun god. Families keep vigil throughout the night, telling stories, reading poetry, eating special foods that represent the warmth of summer, and burning bonfires to ward off the forces of darkness.

Tonight, create your own erotic Winter Solstice celebration that will last throughout the night. Build a fire in the fireplace or light candles, and create a sumptuous winter banquet. Read each other erotic stories or poetry, which you can find on sites like Clean Sheets (www.cleansheets.com) or Nerve.com (www.nerve.com). Stretch out your lovemaking as long as you can, and when you finally do climax, the results will be spectacular. You might even be able to extend your orgasm by continuing to stimulate yourself after your first climax. For him, bring him several times to a four or five on the orgasmic Richter scale before letting him finally explode into a ten. The nights only get shorter from here on out, so make the most of this one.

DECEMBER

Capricorn: Ways to Get Your Goat

If your or your partner's birthday is between December 22 and January 19, you fall under the astrological sign of Capricorn, the Goat. Astrologers consider Capricorns to be responsible, practical, hard-working, and serious, but don't let that fool you. Remember, the symbol for this sign is the goat, traditionally portrayed as the horniest animal in the wild kingdom. In public, your average Capricorn will be the paragon of respectability. Once the bedroom door shuts behind him, watch out.

Your Capricorn man won't need to be wined and dined to get him in the mood. With his strong sex drive, he's willing and anxious to get down to business. He'll appreciate a straightforward (and sexy) overture. Call him at the office and tell him exactly what you'd like to do to him that night. Just make sure he's not on speakerphone—Capricorns prize discretion.

If you're a Capricorn yourself, you want to be the best at everything—including sex. You're eager to try new things and are very solicitous of your man's needs. However, since Capricorns tend to be workaholics, be sure that you let your sexy, fun side peek out once in a while. If you can manage it, grab your man for a weekend out of town, where you can get away from computers, ringing phones, and holiday stress. This time of year, a ski weekend in a quiet mountain cabin could be just the ticket. Once you're in your own private winter wonderland, open a copy of the *Kama Sutra*, light a fire in the fireplace, and prepare to expand your sexual repertoire.

DECEMBER

Position of the Week: A Singing Monkey

According to the Chinese zodiac, people born in the Year of the Monkey are fun, clever, cheerful, and energetic. As you might expect, Monkeys have a lively love life! Approach the position called A Singing Monkey with a sense of humor and fun.

Your man keeps his legs outstretched like a tree branch as you lower yourself onto him in a sitting position. If you need to, you can support yourself by placing a hand on his leg for balance. For a nice treat, have him slide his hands under your butt to help you move on top of him. Encourage him to pull on your cheeks slightly to create a pleasurable taut sensation around your perineum and anus. If you tense your thigh muscles in time with your rocking motion, you'll soon be singing with bliss!

DECEMBER

'Twas the Night Before Ecstasy

Your hands, mouth, and sex aren't the only parts of your body you can use to give him pleasure. Let him slide his penis between your breasts and across your nipples. Cover them with lube or massage oil to make the sensation even more arousing. Press your breasts together around his shaft, and don't be shy about twirling your nipples between your fingers. He'll love to watch.

Another treat for him is a move sometimes referred to as a "back slider" by gay men. Stretch out on your stomach with pillows propped under your hips, or present your beautiful behind to him from a kneeling position, while he adorns your cheeks with lube and proceeds to slide his erection between them. You can also give him some delicious torment by letting him rub his tip between your vaginal lips—but forbid him to slip inside!

Here's another variation you both may enjoy. As you lie on your back, clasp your legs tightly together and let him thrust his lubricated penis between your thighs, moving closer and closer to your lips and clitoris. Keep this up until neither of you can stand it anymore, and then pull him inside you.

DECEMBER

Unwrap Yourself for Christmas!

Merry Christmas! Today, unwrap a present he'll never forget—your body! Striptease is a fine art, but one your man will definitely appreciate. You can play music and put on a sexy show for him, or simply spice up your regular bedtime routine.

No matter what you choose, the key is removing each piece of clothing slowly and provocatively, sliding them over your skin as you leisurely unveil your glowing skin bit by bit. Set your foot on a chair as you roll your stockings over your thighs and down your leg. Peel off your dress or blouse by stretching your arms over your head and thrusting your breasts in his direction. Arch your back like a cat, and make sure to caress your nipples, belly, and sex for his fascinated gaze. For a truly erotic effect, leave on one piece of clothing or jewelry to set off your nudity.

"I love performing stripteases for my boyfriend," says a friend who wants only to be identified as Kiki. "Because I get such a kick out of role-playing and performing, these stripteases often arouse me as much as him! The entire process—from selecting the appropriate song, to deciding what lingerie and makeup to wear, and choreographing my moves—results in a performance that always ends with passionate sex. My man gets so into it that as I'm stripping, he'll slip folded dollar bills into my G-string. What excites me is the look of raw and utter lust on his face. It's completely flattering and invigorating to think that I can be more than his sweet, smart, proper girlfriend."

DECEMBER

Movie Night

As the end of the year approaches, Hollywood studios race to open their films before December 31 so that they qualify for Oscar consideration. Why not have a private screening of your own? Watching an X-rated movie with your man can be an exciting way to turn you both on. Yes, nice women do watch pornography. "I'm a big fan of good, clean porn," says my friend Melissa. "It's particularly arousing when you can tell the actors and actresses are really into it and enjoying what they're doing. To me, porn is a safe, private, and exciting way to add to my sexual experience."

The quality of adult movies has greatly improved and the variety has increased, so don't worry that you'll have to sit through something you find boring or offensive. Your options range from soft-core fare like Showtime's *Red Shoe Diaries* all the way to hard-core flicks. (Many straight women get turned on watching gay porn, so don't rule that genre out.) A new crop of feminist and lesbian producers are making films aimed at both women and couples—films with higher production values, better acting, and decent plots. Look for movies from Candida Royalle's Femme Productions, SIR Videos, or Sex-Positive Productions, or from directors like the highly praised Andrew Blake.

Good Vibrations' Web site (www.goodvibes.com) rates movies according to a variety of criteria, including the quality of the filmmaking and the diversity of the cast. Soon you'll get a feel for where your tastes lie. And when you're screening your selections, keep your man or trusty vibrator nearby, because you never know when you'll want to replicate what's onscreen.

HISTORICAL NOTE: Today is the birthday of author Henry Miller (1891-1980), whose sexually candid autobiographical novel *Tropic of Cancer* was banned from publication in the United States until 1961, even though it was published in France in 1934.

DECEMBER

Japanese Love Hotel

With the stress of the holidays drawing to a close, here's a way for you and your man to relax. Take a cue from Japanese expertise in the art of pampering, and turn your bedroom into a "love hotel." According to Jina Bacarr, author of *The Japanese Art of Sex: How to Tease, Seduce and Pleasure the Samurai in Your Bedroom*, these popular lodgings came about in response to a 1960s curfew barring women in men's hotel rooms after nine p.m. A respectable businessman and his paramour could go to a Western-style hotel, but they risked the gazes and smirks of desk clerks. To save couples embarrassment, the love hotel was born.

"Today, these inns are not just for new lovers," says Bacarr. "They're also for married or committed couples seeking privacy in an overcrowded society. (The phrase *rabu hoteru*, 'love hotel,' is no longer used, but the abbreviation *rabu-ho* and Love Ho are still heard.) These hotels prefer to be known as fashion hotels, couples hotels, boutique hotels, leisure hotels, or theme hotels."

Modern love hotels are fully equipped for pleasure, with vending machines that offer such goodies as dildos, vibrators, and even handcuffs. With this is mind, set up your own display in your bedroom at home, then invite your man in and let him choose which toys he wants to use. If you can find it, try a unique Japanese vibrator called Kuri Kuri (for a chestnut, in honor of its resemblance to the clitoris). He slips the unit over his penis, and when he enters you, the pressure of his body against yours turns the vibrator on. You can also vibrate it directly against your clitoris. Tell him to sit back and watch you pleasure yourself, and soon he'll be saying "*domo arigato*," a special way of saying "thank you" in Japanese!

HISTORICAL NOTE: Marlene Dietrich (1901-92), the actress and sex symbol famous for her "femme fatale" roles and husky voice, was born on this day in Berlin.

DECEMBER

Have Chocolate, Will Orgasm

Chocolate, that staple of so many holiday confections, may not only make you healthier when consumed in small quantities—it may make you hornier, too. Chocolate contains phenylethylamine, a natural component that, according to *Food and Mood* by Elizabeth Somer, stimulates the nervous system, increases blood pressure and heart rate, and "is suspected to produce feelings similar to those experienced when a person is 'in love.'" There's no "suspecting" about it: Lovers have known about the aphrodisiac quality of chocolate for centuries. In her book *All About Chocolate*, Carole Bloom says that Casanova used chocolate to seduce women.

And there's more good news. Eating chocolate releases serotonins into the brain, which helps you feel calm, stabilize your mood, and increase sexual desire. Chocolate also triggers endorphin release, which sends high levels of energy and feelings of euphoria to the brain. It can even increase feelings of self-esteem.

But wait, there's more! Chocolate contains a substance called anandamide, named after the Sanskrit word *ananda*, or bliss. Anandamide helps stimulate and open synapses in the brain, says Bloom. These are the same synapses that respond to marijuana, but, she warns, you'd have to eat more than twenty-five pounds of chocolate in one sitting to get the same high. A single beautiful chocolate truffle will not only make a great snack when you want to take a break from lovemaking: It may just give you that instant charge you need to get and keep you in the mood.

DECEMBER

Eat for Ecstasy

There's no need to fill your pantry with exotic pills and powders in order to keep your body primed for love. Just eat a balanced diet! Foods containing the B vitamins (thiamine, riboflavin, niacin, panthothenic acid, and pyridoxine), such as eggs, milk, nuts, grains, fruit, and veggies, keep your nervous system healthy, which has positive ramifications for your orgasms. Zinc, found in red meat, fish, liver, mushrooms, and grains, is an important component of the enzymes used in sexual function. (Oysters contain lots of zinc, which perhaps accounts for their legendary aphrodisiacal qualities.) In fact, seafood is a good source of protein, which your body needs to keep your sex hormones functioning in tip-top shape. Spice up your meal with chilies, too—your body reacts to the heat by producing endorphins, resulting in a euphoric lover's high. Some research suggests that a small amount of red wine boosts testosterone levels.

If you're looking for libido-boosting remedies to add to your daily smoothie, try Vitamin C for energy, and bee pollen, which some claim will lift not only your energy level but your libido as well. Arginine is often touted as an aphrodisiac, but instead of wasting money on fancy supplements, seek out foods rich in arginine, for example, fish.

Finally, if all else fails, go outside. Get fifteen minutes of sunshine, and your brain will release serotonin, putting you more in the mood for some serious nooky.

HISTORICAL NOTE: Today is the birthday of Jeanne-Antoinette Poisson (1721-64), also known as Madame de Pompadour, the influential mistress of Louis XV of France.

DECEMBER

Position of the Week: Standing Rear Entry

If you're having sex while standing up outdoors or in a public place—say you're in Hawaii watching a beautiful sunset and neither of you wants to miss a moment—try having him enter you from behind as you brace yourself on a balcony railing or other support. This position works great when you're wearing a skirt. All you have to do is lean over slightly, hike up the fabric, and let him start plunging into you.

However, if you don't want to or can't disrobe, you have other sensual options. My lawyer friend Karen describes how her boyfriend made one of her fantasies come true: "I had always wanted to have an orgasm in a public place, in a crowd of people. One year, we went to New York for New Year's Eve. It was cool, but not freezing cold. We joined the throngs at Times Square, and soon found ourselves being pushed closer and closer together. At one point, I was standing behind my boyfriend, pressed up against him, and he reached back, unzipped my jeans, and masturbated me to an orgasm. My coat was open, so he had easy access, and we were so tightly packed that no one could see what was going on. It was probably the most intense, if quiet, orgasm that I have ever had."

How are *you* celebrating New Year's Eve tomorrow?

DECEMBER

New Year's Eve: The Year in Review

We've reached the end of the year, and it's time to take stock. How did you do on meeting your list of sensual resolutions? With a journal or pad of paper in hand, ask yourself the following questions:

- ✦ What sexual activities did you especially enjoy? What would you like to try that you didn't?

- ✦ What new techniques and positions did you try? Were there any that helped bring you to ecstasy over and over again? Why do you think that is?

- ✦ Were you able to accept your sexual self and love your body for all the wonderful sensations it can give you? Why or why not?

- ✦ Were you able to tell your partner exactly what pleases you? What roadblocks, if any, did you have to open communication about your sexuality? How do you think you could knock down those blocks?

- ✦ Did you change any lifestyle habits, such as diet or exercise, that affected your sexual response?

- ✦ What kinds of fantasies did you enjoy? Why do you think that is?

- ✦ How would you describe your orgasms overall?

Remember, your answers are *for your eyes only*. The idea is to learn more about yourself and recognize your accomplishments, not to beat yourself up.

Now that you've taken stock, celebrate the close of the year by doing at least one thing to honor your sexual self. Maybe it's as simple as wearing a piece of lingerie that makes you feel like the Sex Goddess you are, or maybe you want to ring in the New Year by sipping a glass of your favorite champagne and then making slow, tender love to your man. Tonight, it's your choice. See you in the New Year!

ABOUT THE AUTHOR

Cynthia W. Gentry is an award-winning fiction writer, screen-writer, and journalist. She is the co-author, with David Ramsdale, of *Red Hot Tantra: Erotic Secrets of Red Tantra for Intimate Soul-to-Soul Sex and Ecstatic, Enlightened Orgasms.* Her short fiction, essays, and film reviews have appeared in several literary journals and on the Web. She received a bachelor's degree from Stanford University and a master's degree from the University of California at Berkeley's Graduate School of Journalism.